Intermittent Fasting for Beginners

+

Intermittent Fasting for Women Over 60

2 BOOKS IN 1

A Complete Guide for Women to Learn Why It Is Never Too Late to Start Fasting | With Delicious Recipes, 60-Day Meal Plan, 14-Day Exercise Plan & a Journal Diary

By

Melinda Francis

© Copyright 2023 by Melinda Francis- All rights reserved.

The material presented in this work is intended to be both accessible and accurate. The publisher is under no obligation to furnish any accounting, legal, or other services deemed necessary for the purchase or enjoyment of the book. When in doubt, consult an attorney or other knowledgeable expert.

The American Bar Association, the American Publishers Association, and the Trade Associations have approved a Statement of Principles. In relation to this declaration, no part of this book may be duplicated in any way, electronic or physical. It is illegal to make copies of this publication, and you may not keep a copy without the editor's consent. All privileges are protected.

The contents of this document are represented as accurate and consistent, and the reader, whether or not he or she has carefully read it, accepts full responsibility for any damage resulting from the use or misuse of any procedures, instructions, or policies described herein. The publisher of this book assumes no responsibility or liability for any costs incurred as a result of using the information included herein, whether such costs are direct or indirect.

The authors have any and all unclaimed copyrights.

This text is meant solely for educational purposes, and the advice given below is applicable to everyone. There is no agreement or guarantee attached to this material.

Both the publication and the unauthorized use of the trademarks lack the consent and endorsement of the trademark holders. Any brand names or trademarks used herein are for illustrative purposes only. All rights reserved; not related to the content of this text.

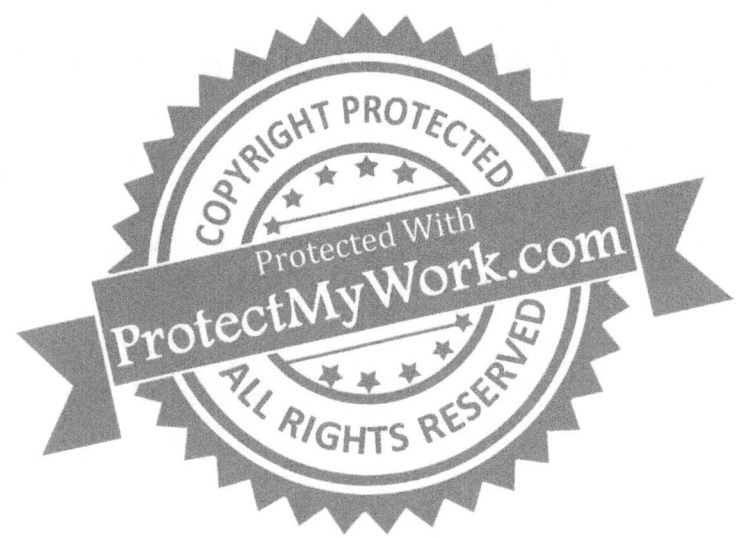

Table of Contents

INTERMITTENT FASTING FOR BEGINNERS 7

Introduction 7

Chapter 1: Understanding Intermittent Fasting 8

    1.1 Exploring Intermittent Fasting Plans 9

    1.2 The Freedom of Choice 9

    1.3 Differentiating From Similar Diets 10

    1.4 Pros And Cons Of Intermittent Fasting 11

Chapter 2: Types of Intermittent Fasting 13

    2.1 Successfully Incorporating Fasting into Your Lifestyle 14

    2.2 How to Start Your Intermittent Fasting Plan 15

    2.3 The Body's Response to Fasting 17

    2.4 How To Face Challenging Days in Intermittent Fasting 19

    2.5 Intermittent Fasting and Meditation 20

Chapter 3: Foods To Eat And Limit On An Intermittent Fasting Diet 22

    3.1 Foods To Eat 22

    3.2 Printable List of Intermittent Fasting Recommended Food Items 23

    3.3 Foods to Limit on an Intermittent Fasting Diet 25

INTERMITTENT FASTING FOR WOMEN OVER 60 26

Chapter 1: Embracing Change and Nurturing Your Well-being 26

    1.1 Recognizing and Embracing Physical Changes 26

    1.2 Health Benefits of Intermittent Fasting for Women Over 60 27

    1.3 Risks of Intermittent Fasting for Women Over 60 29

Chapter 2: Exercise While Fasting 31

    2.1 14-Day Exercise Plan During Intermittent Fasting for Women Over 60 32

    2.2 Tips for Working Out While Intermittent Fasting 34

    2.3 Yoga and Intermittent Fasting: Combining for Optimal Health 35

Chapter 3: Breakfast Recipes For Intermittent Fasting 37

    1. Poached Eggs & Avocado Toasts 37

    2. French Vanilla Almond Granola 38

    3. Baked Potato 38

    5. Vegan Coconut Kefir Banana Muffins 39

    6. Zucchini and Cheese Scrambled Eggs 40

    7. Egg Scramble with Sweet Potatoes 41

8. Spicy Spanish Tomato Baked Eggs 42

9. Smoked Salmon and Avocado Wrap 42

10. Almond Flour Pancakes with Sugar-Free Syrup 43

11. Green Smoothie with Spinach, Kale, and Pineapple 44

12. Chia Seed Pudding with Mixed Berries 44

13. Quinoa Breakfast Bowl with Nuts and Seeds 45

14. Low-Carb Vegetable Omelette 46

15. Greek Yogurt Parfait with Berries and Almonds 46

16. Cinnamon Walnut Baked Apples 47

17. Zucchini and Spinach Egg Muffins 48

18. Broccoli and Cheddar Mini Crustless Quiches 49

19. Blueberry Protein Smoothie 49

20. Vegetable Frittata with Turmeric and Herbs 50

Chapter 4: Lunch Recipes For Intermittent Fasting 51

1. Baked Mahi Mahi 51

2. Sweet Potato and Black Bean Burrito 52

3. Warm Roasted Vegetable Farro Salad 53

4. Roasted Broccoli with Lemon Garlic & Toasted Pine Nuts 54

5. Creamy Black Bean Soup 55

6. Lentil Veggie Burgers 56

7. BBQ Chicken Tostadas 57

8. Buffalo Chicken Sandwich with Blue Cheese Slaw 57

9. Oriental Turkey Burger 58

10. Shrimp Diablo Spaghetti 60

11. Grilled Lemon Herb Salmon 61

12. Greek Chicken Souvlaki with Tzatziki Sauce 62

13. Zucchini Noodles with Pesto and Cherry Tomatoes 63

14. Spicy Thai Shrimp Salad with Peanut Dressing 63

15. Moroccan Chickpea Stew with Quinoa 64

16. Teriyaki Tofu and Vegetable Skewers 65

17. Mediterranean Zoodle Bowl with Olives and Feta 66

18. Lemon Garlic Shrimp and Asparagus Stir-Fry 67

19. Asian Sesame Chicken Salad 68

20. Roasted Vegetable Quinoa Bowl with Tahini Dressing 69

Chapter 5: Dinner Recipes For Intermittent Fasting 70

1. Cajun Potato, Prawn/Shrimp, and Avocado Salad 70

2. Cauliflower Pizza Crust 71

3. Sweet Potato Curry With Spinach And Chickpeas...71
4. Vegan Fried 'Fish' Tacos..72
5. Baked Parmesan Tilapia Delight..73
6. Shredded Brussels Sprouts with Bacon and Onions...74
7. Sauerkraut Salad..75
8. Vegetable Turkey Meatloaf with Balsamic Glaze..76
9. Italian Chicken..77
10. Rustic Shepherd's Pie...78
11. Cauliflower Rice Stir-Fry with Tofu and Vegetables..79
12. Quinoa Stuffed Bell Peppers with Black Beans and Avocado...80
13. Lemon Herb Baked Cod with Steamed Green Beans..81
14. Ratatouille with Herbed Quinoa..81
15. Baked Eggplant Parmesan with Mixed Greens Salad..82
16. Teriyaki Salmon with Sesame Broccoli..83
17. Cilantro Lime Shrimp with Avocado Salsa...84
18. Spinach and Mushroom Stuffed Portobello Mushrooms..84
19. Eggplant and Chickpea Coconut Curry with Brown Rice...85
20. Grilled Steak with Chimichurri Sauce and Roasted Sweet Potatoes...86

Chapter 6: Snack & Dessert Recipes For Intermittent Fasting...87
1. Roasted Cauliflower "Popcorn"...87
2. Spicy Chocolate Keto Fat Bombs...87
3. Citrus Dark Chocolate Mousse..88
4. Peanut Butter Cookies...89
5. Mango and Passionfruit Roulade..90
6. Almond Butter Chocolate Chip Cookies..90
7. Frozen Strawberry-Chocolate Greek Yogurt...91
8. Dark Chocolate Dipped Strawberries..92
9. Pumpkin Spice Protein Bites..93
10. Peanut Butter Banana Bites..93
11. Lemon Coconut Bliss Balls...94
12. Cinnamon Apple Chips...95
13. Raspberry Almond Thumbprint Cookies...95
14. No-Bake Oatmeal Energy Bars...96
15. Chocolate Avocado Pudding..97

60-Day Meal Plan: 16:8 (16 hours fasting, 8 hours eating)..98

Guided Intermittent Fasting Tracker...115

Guided Roadmap for Intermittent Fasting 120

Conclusion 121

INTERMITTENT FASTING FOR BEGINNERS

Introduction

Intermittent fasting has gained popularity in recent years due to its wide range of health benefits and its non-restrictive approach to food choices. Research has shown that fasting can be beneficial for weight loss, mental health improvement, and may even have a protective effect against certain cancers. For women over 60, intermittent fasting can offer additional advantages in terms of preventing muscle, nerve, and joint diseases.

As adults age, practicing intermittent fasting can lead to weight loss and a reduced risk of age-related conditions. A recent study conducted by Baylor College of Medicine revealed that intermittent fasting has the potential to lower blood pressure levels. The study indicated that fasting could achieve this by influencing the gut flora, showcasing the intricate connection between fasting and various aspects of health.

For women over the age of 60, weight loss and overall health improvement become significant concerns. The challenges of losing weight after 60 are often attributed to factors like a decrease in metabolic rate, joint discomfort, reduced muscle mass, and sleep issues. Nevertheless, shedding excess weight, especially harmful abdominal fat, can substantially reduce the risk of developing serious health conditions such as diabetes, heart disease, and cancer.

As we age, the likelihood of facing a variety of health issues increases. In this context, intermittent fasting can serve as a genuine fountain of youth for women over 60, providing effective weight loss solutions and contributing to the prevention of age-related conditions like heart disease and diabetes. By embracing intermittent fasting, women in this age group can embark on a journey towards better health and overall well-being.

Chapter 1: Understanding Intermittent Fasting

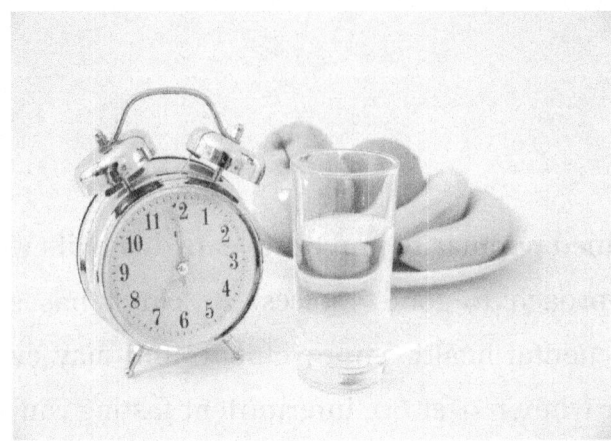

Intermittent fasting, or IF, is a unique eating plan that revolves around alternating between fasting periods and regular mealtimes. Studies suggest that IF can aid in weight management and even potentially reverse certain health conditions.

While many diets focus on what foods to eat, intermittent fasting shifts the focus to when you eat. In other words, you consume your meals within specific time frames. By fasting for designated periods each day or consuming only one meal a couple of days a week, your body can tap into its fat stores for energy. Researchers propose that our bodies have evolved to endure extended periods without food, dating back to the time when early humans were hunters and gatherers.

Maintaining a healthy weight used to be more straightforward in the past. According to Christie Williams, M.S., R.D.N., a nutritionist at Johns Hopkins, factors like limited access to technology, outdoor activities, and less 24/7 entertainment contributed to a healthier lifestyle. However, with the advent of technology and sedentary habits, obesity, heart disease, type 2 diabetes, and other health issues have become prevalent. Intermittent fasting presents a promising approach to counteracting these modern challenges.

Intermittent fasting offers various approaches, but they all share the common principle of defining regular eating and fasting windows. Dr. Mark Mattson, a leading researcher in the field, explains that during fasting, the body eventually exhausts its sugar reserves and transitions to burning fat – a metabolic switch.

Contrasting with the typical American eating habit, where people consume multiple meals and snacks throughout the day, intermittent fasting promotes a more controlled eating schedule. By waiting until your body has burned through the calories from your last meal and starts utilizing fat stores, intermittent fasting can enhance weight loss and overall health.

1.1 Exploring Intermittent Fasting Plans

Before embarking on an intermittent fasting plan, it's crucial to consult your doctor for approval and guidance. Once you receive the green light, the actual practice is relatively simple. One popular approach is the 16/8 fast, where you eat within an eight-hour window and fast for sixteen hours. Many individuals find this daily routine easy to maintain over time. Another option is the "5:2 approach," which involves eating normally for five days a week and reducing calorie intake to 500–600 calories on the other two days. Carefully select your one-meal days, such as Mondays and Thursdays, to adhere to this pattern. However, it's important not to go too long without eating, as prolonged fasting may trigger the body to store extra fat as a survival mechanism. The adjustment period to intermittent fasting may take a couple of weeks, during which you might experience hunger or irritability. Yet, research participants often persist with the strategy, noting improvements in how they feel once they adapt to the new eating pattern.

What to Eat During Intermittent Fasting. During fasting periods, water and zero-calorie drinks like black coffee and tea are acceptable. When it comes to eating, focus on balanced meals with unprocessed carbs, healthy fats, lean protein, whole grains, and leafy greens. The flexibility of intermittent fasting allows for a diverse and enjoyable array of meals, which can be shared with friends and family to enhance the dining experience.

Safety Considerations for Intermittent Fasting. While intermittent fasting can be beneficial for many, it may not be suitable for everyone. Children, teens under 18, pregnant or nursing women, individuals with type 1 diabetes who take insulin, and those with a history of eating disorders should avoid intermittent fasting. For those who fall outside these categories, intermittent fasting can be practiced indefinitely as a positive lifestyle change. However, it's essential to remember that individuals respond differently to intermittent fasting. If you experience any concerning symptoms like anxiety, headaches, or nausea after starting intermittent fasting, consult your doctor for personalized guidance and support.

1.2 The Freedom of Choice

Intermittent fasting (IF) stands out as a distinctive and alluring eating plan among the plethora of diets available today. Unlike most traditional diets that dictate what to eat and what to avoid, intermittent fasting focuses on the "when" rather than the "what" of eating. This novel approach allows for a more flexible and enjoyable eating experience, making it easier to stick with the plan in the long run. One of the most captivating aspects of intermittent fasting is its inclusivity when it comes to food choices. Unlike many diets that restrict certain food categories, IF leaves the decision-making entirely in your hands during the designated feasting periods. There are no forbidden foods; you can enjoy your favorite meals without guilt, provided they are consumed within your eating window. By allowing this level of freedom, intermittent fasting embraces the philosophy of moderation and balance. Caloric restriction can be achieved without having to give up the foods you love. This sense of empowerment contributes to a sustainable and enjoyable eating experience, fostering a positive relationship with food.

Caloric Considerations. When following a time-restricted intermittent fasting plan, you have the opportunity to meet your daily caloric needs during your eating window. Plans such as the 16/8 method or eat/stop/eat provide a 6–8-hour window to ensure adequate caloric intake. However, it's essential to be mindful of other forms of intermittent fasting, like alternate-day fasting or the 5:2 plan, which significantly restrict food intake on fasting days. These methods may not provide enough calories to meet your daily requirements, leading to potential nutrient deficiencies. To ensure you are consuming enough calories for your specific needs, consulting with a healthcare professional or using a calorie calculator is recommended. Balancing your caloric intake and adhering to a well-rounded diet during the eating periods is crucial for overall health and well-being. Intermittent fasting plans do not dictate or exclude any specific food groups. However, on fasting days, it may be challenging to consume the recommended daily intake of various food categories due to limited eating opportunities. For example, following the 5:2 diet may make it difficult to reach the suggested carbohydrate intake, leading to an imbalance in nutrient intake. Moreover, some intermittent fasting regimens advocate total fasting (nearly no calories) on fasting days, which can make it challenging to meet any USDA-recommended consumption guidelines. As with any diet, it is crucial to prioritize balanced nutrition, even during intermittent fasting. Finding creative ways to include a variety of nutrient-rich foods during eating periods ensures that your body receives the essential vitamins, minerals, and macronutrients it needs for optimal health.

1.3 Differentiating From Similar Diets

While intermittent fasting stands out for its unique approach to eating, it is worth understanding how it differs from other popular diets that incorporate periods of dietary restriction. Let's explore some of these diets briefly:

- 3-Day Diet: This plan involves severe calorie restriction for three days, which can lead to temporary weight loss but is unlikely to be sustained. It often lacks essential nutrients, making it challenging to meet recommended dietary guidelines.

- Body Reset Diet: A 15-day diet that focuses on liquid smoothies in the initial phase, followed by the gradual reintroduction of solid foods. While it encourages an active lifestyle, its short duration limits long-term health benefits.

- Fast Diet: A variation of intermittent fasting that involves eating a typical diet five days per week and reducing calorie intake on two days. While it may promote weight loss and potential health improvements, more extensive research is needed to verify its long-term benefits.

- Master Cleanse Lemonade Diet: A rigorous 10-day program centered on lemon-flavored beverages and saltwater intake.

    Severely restricted in calories and nutrients, it may cause health issues and is unlikely to provide lasting weight loss results.

By understanding how intermittent fasting differs from these diets, you can make an informed choice about which eating plan best suits your lifestyle and health goals. Always consult with a healthcare professional before embarking on any significant dietary changes, especially if you have pre-existing health conditions. Embrace the uniqueness of intermittent fasting, tailor it to your needs, and enjoy the freedom it offers in shaping a healthier and more fulfilling relationship with food.

1.4 Pros And Cons Of Intermittent Fasting

If you decide to try intermittent fasting, regardless of the method, it's crucial to concentrate on consuming nourishing meals like leafy greens and organic fruits and vegetables. It's important to remember that consuming processed food at meal times will prevent you from reaping the rewards of intermittent fasting. Like every diet, it has its benefits and drawbacks. Let's talk about the benefits and drawbacks of intermittent fasting.

Pros of Intermittent Fasting:

- **It Can Aid Weight Loss:** As previously mentioned, fasting promotes ketogenesis, which enables your body to use stored fat as fuel rather than glucose. Your Human Growth Hormone (HGH), which is associated with fat reduction and muscle building, is increased by intermittent fasting. In one research using alternate fasting days, patients shed an average of 8% of body fat in just eight weeks!

- **Insulin Resistance is Reduced:** According to research, prediabetics may benefit from intermittent fasting by having lower insulin levels and even better insulin sensitivity. According to one study, fasting considerably lowers blood sugar levels and increases weight reduction in type 2 diabetes patients.

- **It Can Reduce Inflammation:** Chronic inflammation is at the root of almost every modern illness, including heart disease, diabetes, obesity, Alzheimer's, autoimmune disease, and cancer. There is good news, though! According to studies, fasting reduces levels of inflammatory cytokines and systemic inflammation. Additionally, it lessens oxidative stress, aiding your body in fending off dangerous free radicals.

- **It May Reduce the Risk of Developing Heart Disease:** According to studies, intermittent fasting can reduce the number of risk factors for heart disease. For instance, in one study, intermittent fasting reduced body fat, body weight, LDL cholesterol, triglycerides, and blood pressure. Adiponectin, a hormone with potent cardioprotective effects, is also produced in higher amounts during fasts.

- **It Promotes Brain Health:** Fasting does not only benefit your heart; it helps your brain too! According to studies, intermittent fasting raises BDNF levels and may even promote the development of new neurons! Low BDNF is associated with depression as well as cognitive impairment and decline. Fasting's anti-inflammatory effects might prevent Alzheimer's and other neurodegenerative diseases, but more study is required in this area.

- **It is Anti-Aging:** Alterations in gene expression brought on by intermittent fasting promote lifespan and lower the risk of chronic disease. How? Fasting induces autophagy, your body's internal housekeeping system. Your body eliminates old or damaged cells during autophagy and recycles the parts for cellular repair.
- **It Encourages Longevity:** Increased autophagy may slow the aging process and lengthen life. Rats that fasted in one research on animals lived up to 83% longer!

Cons of Intermittent Fasting

- **You Can Still Gain Weight:** Intermittent fasting often results in a reduction in total calorie consumption. This is a crucial factor in the efficacy of intermittent fasting for weight loss. Many become frustrated with yo-yo dieting and switch to fasting to lose weight without worrying about calorie counts. If you overeat within your eating window, you can still risk putting on weight. Intermittent fasting does not permit you to eat piles of fast food. For the best outcomes, choose nutrient-dense meals like organic fruits and vegetables, grass-fed meat, wild seafood, and healthy fats for fuel.
- **There are Side Effects:** Intermittent fasting may have negative impacts on certain people. This is especially the case when beginning intermittent fasting for the first time. As their bodies acclimate to calorie restriction, some people may develop what is known as a "fasting headache." Other potential side effects include digestive issues (including nausea, constipation, diarrhea, & bloating), fatigue, dizziness, irritability, sleep disturbances, malnutrition, and dehydration.
- **It Can Influence Disordered Eating:** Some people may develop harmful eating habits due to the restricted nature of intermittent fasting. For instance, intermittent fasting could cause binge eating when one is not fasting. This is especially true for persons who have a history of eating problems. If you struggle with disordered eating, fasting could be detrimental.

Intermittent Fasting Safety:

Although intermittent fasting has many great health advantages, it's not for everyone. If you have any of the following conditions, discuss intermittent fasting with your doctor before starting.

- Diabetes or difficulty regulating blood glucose levels: Diabetic patients must often eat to check their blood sugar levels. If you have diabetes, intermittent fasting may result in dangerously low blood sugar levels. Intermittent fasting has been shown in studies to reduce blood pressure. Therefore, it may be risky for those with low blood pressure.
- Taking certain drugs: Exercise caution if you take blood pressure, thyroid, or diabetes medications. Fasting will affect their absorption. Many medications should also be taken regularly with meals. Consuming them while fasting may change absorption and heighten negative side effects.
- Underweight: If you are underweight, you will need enough consistent calories

Chapter 2: Types of Intermittent Fasting

Intermittent fasting (IF) comes in various forms, each with its unique approach and potential benefits. Let's explore some of the most popular types of intermittent fasting:

- **5:2 Fasting:** The 5:2 fasting method involves eating normally for five days of the week and then restricting calorie intake on the remaining two days. Men consume around 600 calories, while women limit their intake to 500 calories on fasting days. The flexibility of choosing fasting days makes it easier for individuals to comply with this approach. However, caution is advised for those engaging in vigorous endurance exercise during fasting days, as it might impact performance. If you have a training schedule or specific fitness goals, it's best to consult a sports nutritionist before adopting this method.

- **Time-Restricted Fasting:** Time-restricted fasting involves selecting a daily eating window, leaving a fasting period of 14 to 16 hours. Autophagy, the body's cellular cleansing process, is activated during fasting, which can enhance fat metabolism and improve insulin function. You can customize your eating window, such as eating from 9 a.m. to 5 p.m. This method might be suitable for individuals with families who have late dinners, as most of the fasting time occurs during sleep. However, if your schedule is unpredictable, daily periods of fasting might not be the best fit.

- **Overnight Fasting:** The simplest form of IF is overnight fasting, where you fast for 12 hours every day. For instance, you stop eating after dinner at 7 p.m. and resume eating with breakfast at 7 a.m. the next morning. While some autophagy occurs after 12 hours, the cellular benefits are less significant compared to longer fasting periods. This approach is easy to follow and does not require you to skip any meals, just avoid a nightly snack if you had one. However, it may not maximize the benefits of fasting, especially if your goal is weight loss.

- **Eat Stop Eat:** Created by author Brad Pilon, this approach emphasizes flexibility and temporary fasting from eating. The method involves committing to resistance training and executing one or two 24-hour fasts per week. After the fast, individuals can return to their regular eating routine without the need for strict diets. The focus is on avoiding binge eating after fasting and maintaining a balanced approach to eating. Combining regular exercise with occasional fasting can result in a calorie deficit without feeling restricted.

- **Whole-Day Fasting:** With whole-day fasting, you eat only one meal a day, typically dinner, and then fast until the next day's dinner or lunch. While this approach makes it difficult to consume all daily calories at once, it might be challenging to get all necessary nutrients in one meal. Also, hunger pangs during the day could lead to poor food choices during the meal, impacting overall nutrition intake.

- **Alternate-Day Fasting:** Popularized by nutrition professor Krista Varady, alternate-day fasting involves fasting every other day, consuming only 25% of daily caloric needs on fasting days. Studies have shown significant reductions in body mass index, weight, and cholesterol in obese individuals following this method. While hunger-related negative effects tend to subside over time, some individuals might find it challenging to maintain this strategy due to never feeling fully satiated on fasting days.
- **Choose-Your-Day Fasting:** This flexible IF approach allows individuals to choose when to practice time-restricted fasting, whether every other day or once or twice a week. It's akin to occasionally skipping breakfast or adjusting eating times to fit your schedule. While this method offers more flexibility, the results might be milder compared to more structured fasting approaches.

It's important to remember that the effectiveness of intermittent fasting varies from person to person. Finding the right method that aligns with your lifestyle and health goals is key to a successful and sustainable intermittent fasting experience. If you have any medical conditions or concerns, consult with a healthcare professional before starting any fasting regimen.

2.1 Successfully Incorporating Fasting into Your Lifestyle

Fasting, an age-old practice of food restriction, has gained popularity for its numerous benefits related to longevity, health, and weight loss. Although it may seem challenging to resist the body's natural urge to eat while fasting, it is worth noting that our ancestors, living a hunter-gatherer lifestyle, often endured extended periods of fasting. However, in the modern hectic lifestyle, adopting fasting can still pose certain challenges due to its demanding nature. There are different types of fasting, each with its positive health effects, such as weight loss, protection against conditions like diabetes, cardiovascular diseases, cancers, and even an extended lifespan. Some fasting techniques range from casual meal skipping to more extreme 36-hour prolonged fasts.

One popular method is intermittent fasting (IF), which involves alternating between regular fasting and eating, making it easy to fit into busy schedules since it does not impose strict dietary restrictions during eating windows.

Among the various forms of intermittent fasting, the 5:2 diet allows individuals to restrict caloric intake for two days a week while eating normally on the remaining days. Alternatively, the one meal a day fast (OMAD) or "Warrior fast" involves consuming only one substantial meal daily, and Time Restricted Eating (TRE) includes alternating between fasting and feasting windows throughout the day. TRE offers flexibility, ranging from a simple 12:12 fast (12 hours fasting, 12 hours eating) to a more challenging 20:4 fast (20 hours fasting, 4 hours eating). A popular TRE method is the 16:8, involving 16 hours of fasting at night and 8 hours of eating during the day, following the body's natural circadian rhythm. Since most individuals naturally fast during sleep, extending this fast by a few hours in the morning and evening can easily achieve the 16:8 method. For beginners, it is advisable to avoid extremely prolonged fasts and experiment with different fasting techniques to find the one that best suits their lifestyle.

Unlike fad diets, fasting promotes sustainable weight loss by subjecting the body to food stress, which triggers the metabolic state of ketosis (fat burning).

Setting realistic goals is crucial when incorporating fasting into your lifestyle. While calorie restriction can lead to long-term weight loss by inducing the metabolic state of ketosis, pushing the body too hard can result in weariness and mental exhaustion, counteracting the positive effects of fasting. It is essential to align fasting goals with long-term weight loss objectives and gradually increase fasting windows or frequency to a comfortable level. Starting with a more manageable intermittent fasting goal, like a 12-hour fast once a week, can serve as a better compromise and pave the way for longer fasting durations. To avoid distractions from thoughts of food during fasting, preparation is key. Scheduling your fast around social events and creating a shopping list and cooking plan can ensure wholesome and satisfying meals are available when breaking the fast. Opting for a healthy diet, such as the traditional Mediterranean diet, with fish protein, low glycemic carbohydrates from vegetables, and healthy fats from olive oil, complements fasting and keeps you fuller for longer with fewer calories. Moderation is essential, and occasional indulgence in favorite meals and snacks during feasting hours can help maintain commitment to the fast. Controlling portion sizes and incorporating intermittent fasting into your exercise routine can reduce hunger and prevent overeating. While engaging in vigorous activity during fasting is not recommended, gentle cardiovascular exercises like yoga and walking, as well as short strength-based workouts, can enhance the health benefits of fasting while keeping the body and mind active and curbing food cravings.

Finally, sharing your fasting objectives with friends or colleagues can provide support and accountability. This support system can help you stay on track and may even inspire others to adopt a fasting lifestyle. By following these steps and finding the fasting method that fits your lifestyle, you can successfully incorporate fasting into your daily routine and reap its many health benefits.

2.2 How to Start Your Intermittent Fasting Plan

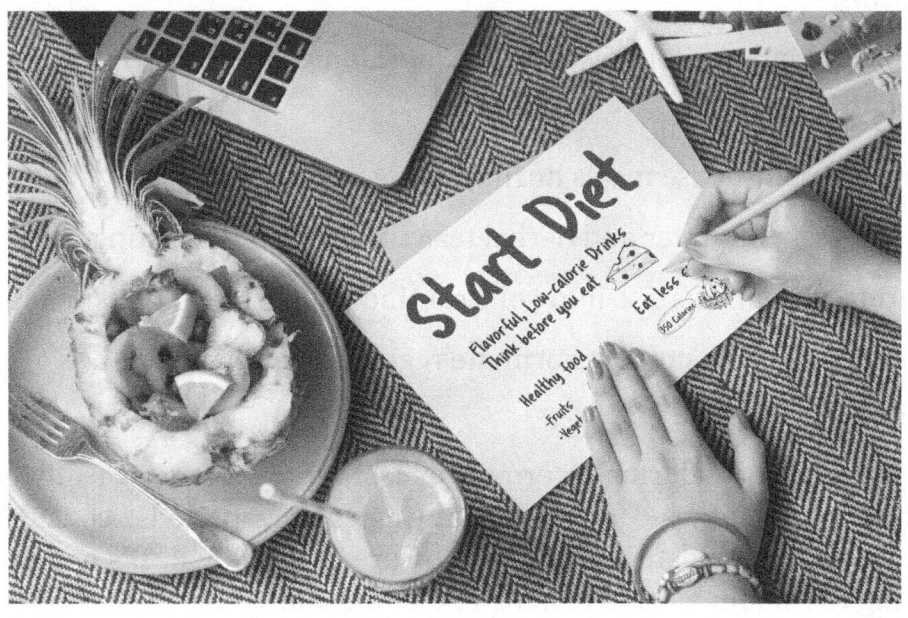

Starting an intermittent fasting plan can be both exciting and challenging. It requires careful consideration of individual preferences, lifestyle, and health goals. In this chapter, we will explore step-by-step guidelines on how to embark on your intermittent fasting journey, tailored to different types of individuals.

Assess Your Lifestyle and Goals

Before diving into intermittent fasting, take some time to evaluate your current lifestyle, daily routines, and health objectives. Consider your work schedule, social commitments, and exercise habits. Are you looking to lose weight, improve energy levels, or enhance overall well-being? Understanding your motivations and lifestyle will help you choose the most suitable fasting approach.

Types of Intermittent Fasting

As discussed earlier, there are various types of intermittent fasting, each with its unique fasting and eating windows. For beginners, it is recommended to start with a less restrictive approach and gradually progress to longer fasting periods if desired. Some popular options include:

- 16:8 method (fasting for 16 hours and eating within an 8-hour window).
- 5:2 diet (eating normally for five days and limiting calories on two non-consecutive days).
- Eat-Stop-Eat (occasional 24-hour fasting days).
- Time-Restricted Eating (adjusting fasting and eating windows throughout the day).
- Ease into Intermittent Fasting

For some individuals, jumping straight into a rigorous fasting schedule may be overwhelming. Consider easing into intermittent fasting by gradually extending your fasting window over a week or two. Start with a 12-hour fast and increase by an hour each day until you reach your desired fasting duration.

Build Good Habits

To support a successful intermittent fasting plan, develop good habits that align with your goals.

These may include:

- Prioritizing nutrient-dense meals during eating windows.
- Staying hydrated with water and herbal teas throughout the fasting period.
- Incorporating regular exercise into your routine to boost metabolism and overall health.
- Getting enough sleep to support hormone regulation and recovery.

Listen to Your Body

As I said many times before, during intermittent fasting, it is crucial to listen to your body's signals. If you feel overly fatigued or unwell during fasting periods, consider adjusting your fasting schedule or seeking guidance from a healthcare professional. It's essential to ensure that intermittent fasting is sustainable and beneficial for your individual needs.

Customize Your Fasting Plan

Intermittent fasting is not a one-size-fits-all approach. Customize your fasting plan to suit your preferences and daily life. For example:

- Busy Professionals: Consider the 16:8 method, as it can easily fit into a standard workday.
- Night Owls: Opt for Time-Restricted Eating with a later eating window that accommodates your natural sleep-wake cycle.
- Fitness Enthusiasts: Try the Eat-Stop-Eat approach to incorporate fasting days around your workout schedule.

Monitor Progress and Adjust

As you start your intermittent fasting plan, regularly monitor your progress and make adjustments as needed. Pay attention to how your body responds to fasting and eating windows. If certain fasting methods do not align with your lifestyle or goals, don't hesitate to try a different approach.

Embarking on an intermittent fasting plan requires thoughtful consideration of personal preferences and lifestyle. By choosing a suitable fasting method, building good habits, and listening to your body, you can create a successful and sustainable intermittent fasting journey that aligns with your health and well-being goals. Remember to be patient with yourself as you adapt to this new lifestyle, and feel free to experiment with different approaches until you find what works best for you.

2.3 The Body's Response to Fasting

Fasting, particularly intermittent fasting, triggers a range of physiological responses in the body. Understanding how the body reacts to different types of intermittent fasting, as well as the role of hormones, weight loss, and physical exercise, can provide valuable insights into the benefits and challenges of this dietary approach.

Hormonal Response to Fasting

Hormones play a crucial role in regulating various bodily functions, and their response to fasting is central to understanding its effects. One of the key hormones affected by intermittent fasting is insulin. When you fast, insulin levels decrease, allowing the body to tap into stored fat for energy. This process, known as ketosis, is a metabolic state in which the body predominantly utilizes fat as its primary energy source. In addition to insulin, other hormones, such as growth hormone (GH) and norepinephrine, are also influenced by fasting. GH levels increase during fasting, promoting fat burning and muscle preservation. Norepinephrine, a hormone that stimulates the breakdown of fat cells, also rises, contributing to enhanced fat utilization during fasting periods. Moreover, fasting affects hormones related to hunger and satiety. Ghrelin, often referred to as the "hunger hormone," increases during fasting, signaling the brain that it is time to eat. On the other hand, leptin, the "satiety hormone," tends to decrease, potentially leading to increased appetite after fasting periods. These hormonal changes can impact eating behaviors and the ability to adhere to fasting protocols.

Weight Loss and Fasting

Intermittent fasting can be an effective tool for weight loss due to its impact on caloric restriction and metabolic processes. By reducing the eating window and fasting for extended periods, individuals naturally consume fewer calories, creating a calorie deficit that promotes weight loss.

Furthermore, the metabolic shift towards ketosis during fasting can enhance fat burning. As the body relies on stored fat for energy, fat cells are broken down, leading to a reduction in body fat. Combined with the preservation of muscle mass through increased GH levels, intermittent fasting can promote a more favorable body composition during weight loss.

It is essential to note that sustainable weight loss through fasting requires a balanced and nutrient-dense diet during the eating windows. Overcompensating with high-calorie, unhealthy foods can negate the benefits of fasting and hinder weight loss progress.

Exercise and Fasting

The role of exercise during fasting is a subject of interest and debate. While engaging in vigorous exercise during fasting may not be advisable due to the potential risk of low energy levels, milder forms of physical activity can complement intermittent fasting.

Gentle cardiovascular exercises like walking, yoga, and light aerobics can be beneficial during fasting periods, as they do not overly strain the body. These activities can help maintain energy levels, promote blood circulation, and support overall well-being.

Strength-based workouts, such as resistance training, can also be incorporated into fasting routines. These exercises stimulate muscle growth and help preserve muscle mass, especially when combined with increased GH levels during fasting. Maintaining muscle mass is crucial for an efficient metabolism and long-term weight management.

However, it is essential to listen to your body during fasting and exercise. If you experience extreme fatigue or dizziness, it may be best to rest and postpone vigorous workouts until after eating periods. Hydration is also crucial during fasting and exercise, as dehydration can exacerbate feelings of fatigue and hinder performance.

The Adaptation Process

As with any dietary change, the body requires time to adapt to intermittent fasting. Initially, individuals may experience hunger pangs, irritability, and difficulty concentrating. These symptoms are normal during the adjustment period.

However, over time, the body becomes more efficient at utilizing stored fat for energy, and hunger hormones may become more manageable. Many individuals report feeling more energized and mentally alert during fasting periods as the body adapts to this metabolic shift.

Moreover, intermittent fasting is a highly individualized approach, and what works for one person may not suit another. Experimenting with different fasting protocols and finding the one that aligns with personal preferences and lifestyle is essential for long-term adherence and success.

In conclusion, the body's response to intermittent fasting involves significant hormonal changes, metabolic adaptations, and potential weight loss benefits. By understanding these responses and incorporating appropriate exercise, individuals can optimize the benefits of intermittent fasting while maintaining a healthy and balanced lifestyle. As with any dietary change, it is crucial to consult with a healthcare professional before embarking on an intermittent fasting journey to ensure it aligns with individual health needs and goals.

2.4 How To Face Challenging Days in Intermittent Fasting

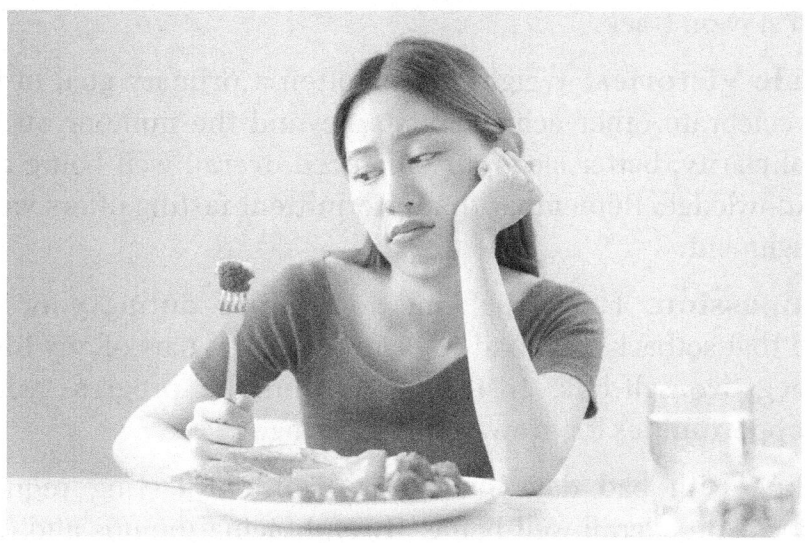

Intermittent fasting is a powerful and beneficial approach to nutrition, but like any lifestyle change, it can present challenges, especially on days when things don't go as planned. Whether it's an unexpected social event, increased stress, or simply feeling low on energy, dealing with bad days during intermittent fasting is essential for maintaining consistency and long-term success.

Embrace Flexibility. One of the key aspects of intermittent fasting is its adaptability. It's essential to recognize that occasional deviations from your fasting schedule are entirely normal and shouldn't be a cause for guilt or frustration. Embrace flexibility and understand that life's unpredictability may occasionally disrupt your fasting routine. Instead of dwelling on a bad day, focus on getting back on track the next day.

Listen to Your Body. While intermittent fasting can offer numerous benefits, it's crucial to listen to your body's cues. If you're feeling unwell, overly fatigued, or exceptionally hungry on a fasting day, don't hesitate to adjust your plan. Consider shifting to a less restrictive fasting method or opting for a smaller eating window. Prioritizing your well-being is crucial for maintaining a positive relationship with intermittent fasting.

Mindful Eating on Non-Fasting Days. On non-fasting days, it's tempting to indulge in large meals or unhealthy foods as a way to compensate for the fasting periods. However, this behavior can lead to overeating and sabotage your progress. Instead, practice mindful eating and choose nutrient-dense foods to nourish your body. Remember that intermittent fasting is not a license to overindulge; it's a sustainable approach to overall health and well-being.

Plan Ahead for Social Events. Social gatherings and events can be tricky to navigate while fasting, but with proper planning, it's manageable. If you know you have an event coming up, consider adjusting your fasting schedule or plan your eating window accordingly. Be mindful of what you consume during the event and opt for healthier choices when possible. Additionally, staying hydrated can help you feel more satiated and reduce the temptation to overeat.

Seek Support and Accountability. Having a support system can significantly impact your success with intermittent fasting. Share your journey with friends, family, or online communities who understand and embrace intermittent fasting. Surrounding yourself with like-minded individuals can provide motivation and encouragement, making it easier to cope with challenging days and stay on track.

Focus on Non-Scale Victories. Weight loss is often a primary goal of intermittent fasting, but it's essential to celebrate other achievements beyond the number on the scale. Improved energy levels, mental clarity, better sleep, or enhanced overall well-being are all valuable non-scale victories to acknowledge. Remember that intermittent fasting offers various health benefits beyond weight management.

Practice Self-Compassion. Lastly, be kind to yourself during your intermittent fasting journey. Understand that setbacks and bad days are a natural part of any lifestyle change. Avoid self-criticism and negative self-talk. Instead, focus on the progress you've made and use challenging days as opportunities for growth and learning.

In conclusion, dealing with bad days during intermittent fasting requires flexibility, self-compassion, and a focus on overall well-being. By embracing the ups and downs of the journey and staying committed to your goals, intermittent fasting can become a sustainable and fulfilling part of your lifestyle.

2.5 Intermittent Fasting and Meditation

In recent years, both intermittent fasting and meditation have gained popularity as powerful practices for improving physical, mental, and emotional well-being. While they may seem unrelated at first glance, these two practices can complement each other and create a harmonious synergy, enhancing the overall benefits of each.

The Connection Between Intermittent Fasting and Meditation

At their core, both intermittent fasting and meditation involve self-discipline and mindfulness. Intermittent fasting requires individuals to be conscious of their eating patterns and make intentional decisions about when to eat and when to fast. On the other hand, meditation cultivates awareness of thoughts and emotions, encouraging individuals to be present in the moment and observe without judgment.

Enhancing Mindfulness in Eating

One of the challenges in intermittent fasting is maintaining mindfulness during eating windows. It's easy to fall into the trap of mindless eating, especially after a period of fasting. Incorporating meditation into mealtime can help foster a deeper sense of mindfulness in eating.

By taking a few moments to meditate before a meal, individuals can become more attuned to their hunger cues, enjoy the sensory experience of eating, and recognize when they are genuinely full.

Managing Stress and Cravings

Stress and food cravings are common challenges during intermittent fasting. Meditation is a powerful tool for managing stress and reducing cravings. Regular meditation practice has been shown to decrease cortisol levels, the stress hormone, which can help individuals stay calm and focused during fasting periods. Additionally, mindfulness meditation can increase self-awareness and emotional regulation, reducing the likelihood of succumbing to impulsive food cravings.

Improving Adherence to Intermittent Fasting

Consistency is key to the success of intermittent fasting. However, it can be challenging to stick to a fasting routine, especially when facing external pressures or temptations to deviate from the plan. Meditation can play a crucial role in improving adherence to intermittent fasting by enhancing willpower, self-control, and the ability to stay committed to the fasting schedule.

Promoting Mind-Body Connection

Both intermittent fasting and meditation promote a stronger mind-body connection. Intermittent fasting allows individuals to become more attuned to their body's hunger and satiety signals, fostering a deeper understanding of their nutritional needs. Meditation, on the other hand, encourages individuals to be present in their bodies, observe bodily sensations, and cultivate a sense of inner peace and acceptance.

Reducing Emotional Eating

Emotional eating is a common obstacle to successful weight management. Many individuals turn to food as a coping mechanism for stress, anxiety, or emotional distress. Through meditation, individuals can develop healthier coping strategies and learn to address emotional triggers without turning to food. This can support the overall success of intermittent fasting by reducing the likelihood of emotional eating during fasting and eating windows.

Enhancing Overall Well-Being

Ultimately, the combination of intermittent fasting and meditation can lead to enhanced overall well-being. By fostering mindfulness, stress reduction, and a deeper mind-body connection, individuals may experience improved physical health, mental clarity, emotional balance, and a greater sense of inner peace.

Integrating meditation into an intermittent fasting routine can amplify the benefits of both practices, creating a synergistic effect on physical and mental health. By cultivating mindfulness, managing stress, and strengthening self-discipline, individuals can enhance their journey towards a healthier and more balanced lifestyle.

Chapter 3: Foods To Eat And Limit On An Intermittent Fasting Diet

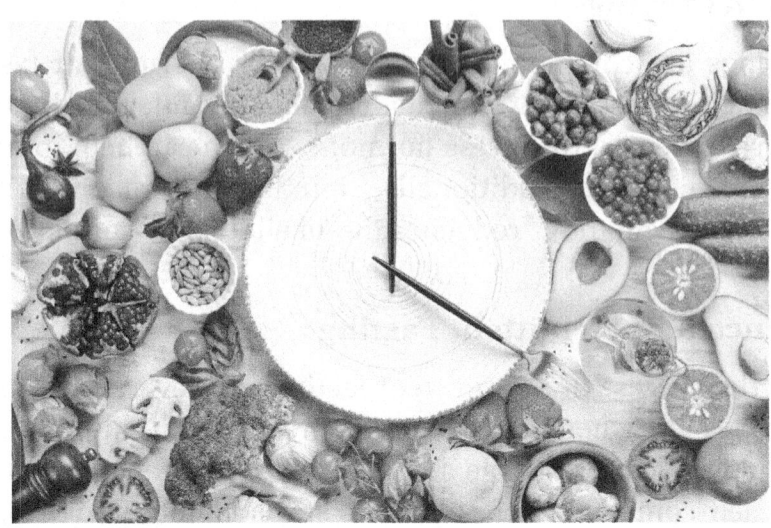

3.1 Foods To Eat

On an intermittent fasting (IF) diet, it is crucial to focus on consuming nutrient-dense foods that provide sustenance and support overall health. Lean proteins play a vital role in helping you feel full for longer periods and preserving or building muscle. Some examples of healthy, lean protein sources include plain Greek yogurt, chicken breast, fish, shellfish, beans, lentils, tofu, and tempeh. Incorporating a variety of fruits and vegetables is essential in any diet plan, including intermittent fasting.

These natural foods are rich in vitamins, minerals, phytonutrients, and fiber, which contribute to intestinal health, blood sugar regulation, and cholesterol reduction. Additionally, they are low in calories, making them an excellent choice for those practicing IF. Some recommended fruits to include in your diet while intermittent fasting are apricots, apples, blackberries, blueberries, cherries, pears, plums, peaches, melons, and oranges.

Vegetables are a crucial component of an IF regimen, and incorporating leafy greens can have significant health benefits. Diets high in leafy greens have been associated with a reduced risk of heart disease, cancer, type 2 diabetes, cognitive decline, and other illnesses. The 2020-2025 Dietary Guidelines for Americans recommend that most adults should consume 2.5 cups of vegetables per day for a 2,000-calorie diet.

Affordable vegetables that can be included in an IF protocol are broccoli, carrots, cauliflower, tomatoes, and green beans. Leafy greens like arugula, spinach, kale, cabbage, chard, and collard greens are excellent choices for their nutrient-rich content and high fiber.

3.2 Printable List of Intermittent Fasting Recommended Food Items

Please note that this list is not exhaustive, and you can add or modify the items based on your personal preferences and dietary requirements. It's essential to choose nutrient-dense and whole foods that support your health and intermittent fasting goals.

Lean Proteins:
- Chicken breast
- Turkey
- Fish (salmon, tuna, cod, etc.)
- Shellfish (shrimp, crab, mussels, etc.)
- Lean cuts of beef or pork
- Eggs
- Tofu and tempeh

Fruits:
- Apples
- Berries (blueberries, strawberries, raspberries, etc.)
- Citrus fruits (oranges, grapefruits, lemons, etc.)
- Apricots
- Pears
- Peaches
- Plums
- Melons (watermelon, cantaloupe, honeydew)

Vegetables:
- Broccoli
- Cauliflower
- Spinach
- Kale
- Tomatoes
- Carrots
- Bell peppers
- Cucumbers
- Zucchini
- Green beans

Healthy Fats:
- Avocado
- Nuts (almonds, walnuts, pistachios, etc.)
- Seeds (chia seeds, flaxseeds, pumpkin seeds, etc.)
- Olive oil
- Coconut oil
- Avocado oil

Beverages:
- Water (plain or infused with fruits/herbs)
- Herbal teas (peppermint, chamomile, ginger, etc.)
- Black coffee (without added sugar or cream)
- Green tea

Condiments and Spices:
- Fresh herbs (parsley, basil, cilantro, etc.)
- Garlic and ginger
- Turmeric
- Cinnamon
- Chili flakes
- Mustard
- Apple cider vinegar

Healthy Carbohydrates:
- Sweet potatoes
- Quinoa
- Brown rice
- Oats (steel-cut or rolled)
- Whole-grain bread (in moderation)
- Lentils
- Chickpeas

Dairy (if tolerated):
- Greek yogurt (plain, unsweetened)
- Cottage cheese

Non-Dairy Alternatives:
- Almond milk (unsweetened)
- Coconut milk (unsweetened)

Healthy Snacks:
- Raw nuts and seeds (portion-controlled)
- Nut butter (almond, peanut, etc.)
- Hummus with raw vegetables
- Rice cakes (whole-grain)
- Popcorn (air-popped, without added butter or excessive salt)

Low-Calorie Foods:
- Cabbage
- Cauliflower rice
- Zucchini noodles (zoodles)
- Mushrooms
- Brussels sprouts

Probiotic Foods:
- Kimchi
- Sauerkraut
- Yogurt with live cultures (if tolerated)

Remember to be mindful of portion sizes and balance your meals with a variety of nutrient-dense foods. It's essential to listen to your body's hunger and fullness cues and make adjustments as needed. Please consult with a healthcare professional or a registered dietitian if you have specific dietary concerns or medical conditions.

3.3 Foods to Limit on an Intermittent Fasting Diet

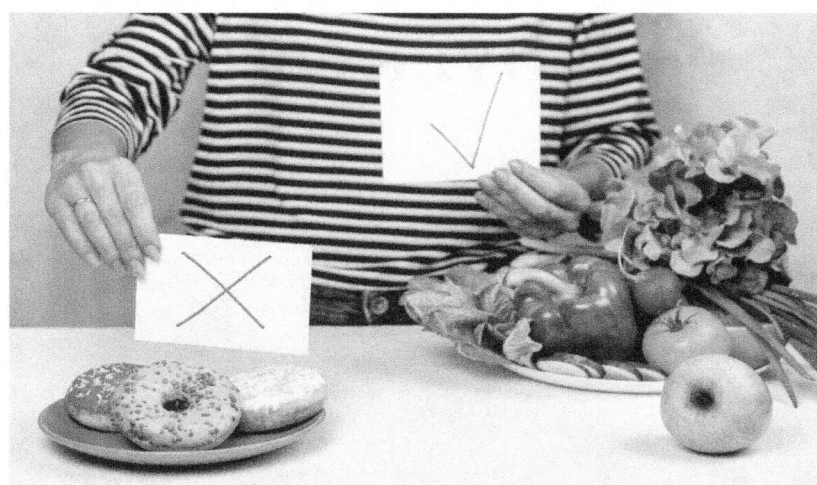

While following an intermittent fasting plan, it is essential to avoid certain types of food that are high in calories, saturated fats harmful to heart health, and excessive salt. Such foods do not provide satiety and can even trigger hunger, defeating the purpose of intermittent fasting. Moreover, they offer little to no nutritional value.

Limit the following foods to maintain a healthy and effective intermittent fasting schedule:

- Snack chips and other processed snacks high in unhealthy fats and calories.
- Pretzels and crackers, which often lack nutritional value and may contain unhealthy additives.
- Meals that contain a significant amount of added sugar. Processed sugars provide empty calories and little to no nutritional benefit, leading to quick metabolism and hunger.
- Examples of sugary foods to avoid during intermittent fasting include candies, cakes, cookies, highly sweetened coffee and teas, fruit drinks, and sugary cereals with little fiber and granola.

By being mindful of the foods you consume and focusing on nutrient-dense options, intermittent fasting can be a more effective and sustainable dietary approach, supporting your overall health and well-being. Remember to consult with a healthcare professional or nutritionist to ensure that intermittent fasting is appropriate for your individual needs and health conditions.

INTERMITTENT FASTING FOR WOMEN OVER 60

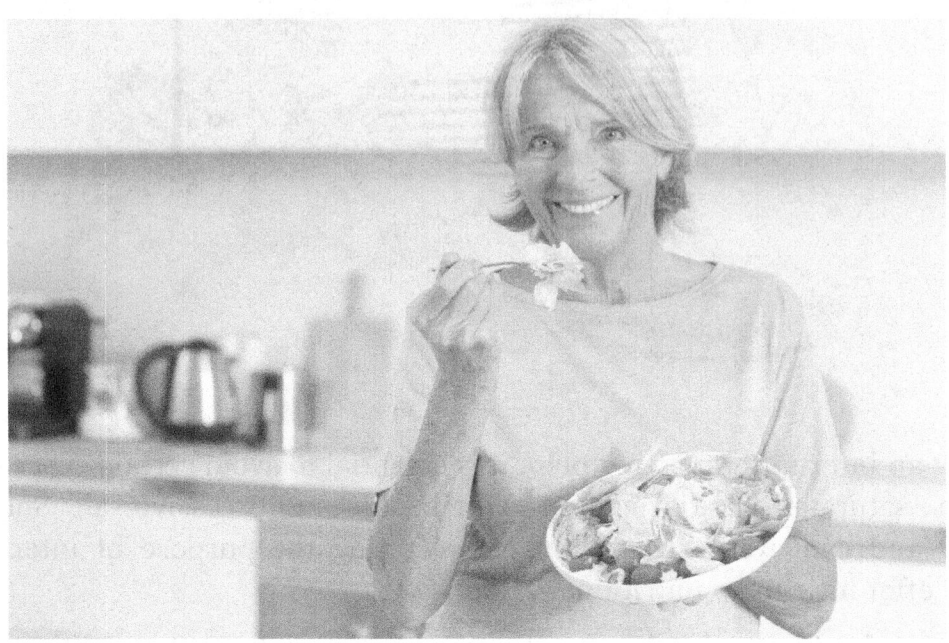

Chapter 1: Embracing Change and Nurturing Your Well-being

As we age, our bodies undergo natural changes that may present certain challenges. However, understanding these changes and proactively caring for ourselves can lead to a fulfilling and healthy life. Embracing the physical changes that come with age and adopting good habits can greatly contribute to overall well-being. In this chapter, we will explore ways to start your journey towards optimal health and happiness as you age gracefully.

1.1 Recognizing and Embracing Physical Changes

Change is an inevitable part of life, and our bodies are no exception. As we grow older, certain bodily systems may experience changes that can affect our daily lives. It is essential to recognize and embrace these changes as a natural part of the aging process. Understanding that these changes are normal can help alleviate any anxiety or concerns that may arise. One of the most noticeable changes occurs in the cardiovascular system. Arteries and the heart may become less flexible, resulting in higher blood pressure. Engaging in a nutritious diet and regular aerobic exercise can support your cardiovascular health and help maintain vitality.

Lungs may also lose some elasticity with age, making breathing more challenging for some individuals. Avoiding smoking and staying active through regular aerobic activity can enhance lung health and promote overall well-being.

The immune system may become less effective as we age, increasing the risk of illnesses. Vaccines, a balanced diet, regular exercise, and other healthy lifestyle choices can help support and strengthen the immune system, reducing the chances of getting sick.

Nurturing Your Body and Mind

Caring for your body and mind is essential at any age, but it becomes even more crucial as you grow older. A holistic approach to well-being can significantly impact your quality of life. Strength training, or resistance training, is a powerful way to maintain and build muscle tone. Coupled with a nutritious diet, it can help reduce body fat and enhance overall muscular health. Prioritizing regular exercise can also help combat age-related muscle loss. Ensuring proper eye and ear health is vital. Regular check-ups with eye doctors and audiologists can help detect any age-related changes in vision and hearing early on, allowing for timely intervention and better management. Routine dental checkups are essential for oral health, as older adults may experience problems such as cavities and gum disease. Early diagnosis and treatment can prevent more severe issues like tooth loss and mouth cancer.

The Importance of Skincare

As our skin undergoes changes with age, it's essential to implement a skincare routine that caters to its specific needs. Skin may become drier, thinner, and more prone to wrinkling. Embracing proper skincare practices, such as using moisturizers and sunscreen, can help protect and nourish the skin. Taking vitamin D supplements, especially if the body's ability to produce vitamin D decreases, can aid in preventing vitamin D insufficiency.

The Gift of Aging

Aging is a privilege and an opportunity to cherish the gift of life. While we cannot change the past, we can embrace the present and make the most of our current circumstances. Cultivating a positive mindset and self-compassion can foster resilience and enable us to navigate life's changes with grace.

Staying active, eating healthily, and taking care of our overall well-being are essential components of aging gracefully. Embracing the physical changes that come with age and nurturing our bodies and minds are acts of self-love that can lead to a fulfilling and happy life at any age.

1.2 Health Benefits of Intermittent Fasting for Women Over 60

Intermittent fasting not only offers weight management benefits but also plays a significant role in reducing the risk of developing chronic diseases for women over 60.

Heart Health

Research has indicated that intermittent fasting can have a positive impact on heart health. In a study involving obese men and women, an eight-week intermittent fasting regimen resulted in a 6 percent reduction in blood pressure. Additionally, the study found a decrease of 25 percent in LDL cholesterol and 32 percent in triglycerides.

While the correlation between intermittent fasting and improved LDL cholesterol levels and triglycerides is not entirely consistent, higher-quality studies are required to better understand its effects on heart health.

Diabetes Management

Intermittent fasting has also shown promise in controlling and reducing the risk of diabetes. By reducing insulin levels and improving insulin resistance, intermittent fasting helps lower some risk factors for diabetes, similar to constant calorie restriction. However, it's essential to note that intermittent fasting might not be equally effective for women as it is for men in terms of blood sugar regulation. Although men's blood sugar remained unaffected, a small study found that women experienced worsened blood sugar regulation after 22 days of alternate-day fasting. Nonetheless, the reduction in insulin and insulin resistance still holds the potential to decrease the risk of diabetes, particularly for individuals with pre-diabetes.

Weight Loss

Intermittent fasting, when done correctly, can be a rapid and effective method for weight loss. The practice of daily short-term fasting can help reduce calorie intake and facilitate weight loss. Numerous studies have shown that intermittent fasting is as effective as traditional calorie-restricted diets for short-term weight loss. For overweight adults, one study revealed an average weight loss of 15 lbs (6.8 kg) over 3-12 months with intermittent fasting. Another review demonstrated a body weight reduction of 3-8 percent in overweight or obese adults over 3-24 weeks, accompanied by a 3-7 percent decrease in waist circumference.

Note: The long-term effects of intermittent fasting on weight loss for women are yet to be fully explored. While intermittent fasting is likely to aid in weight loss, individual results may vary depending on calorie consumption during non-fasting periods and adherence to the lifestyle.

Other Health Benefits

Intermittent fasting has shown potential for providing additional health benefits:

- **Reduced inflammation:** Studies suggest that intermittent fasting can lower key inflammation markers, which may help combat weight gain and various health issues associated with chronic inflammation.

- **Improved psychological well-being:** Research indicates that intermittent fasting can lead to reduced depression and binge eating habits, while also enhancing body image in obese adults after eight weeks of practice.

- **Increased longevity:** While intermittent fasting has been observed to increase the lifespan of rats and mice by 33-83%, its effect on human longevity requires further investigation.

- **Preserved muscle mass:** In comparison to constant calorie restriction, intermittent fasting appears to be more efficient in maintaining muscle mass. Higher muscle mass allows for increased calorie consumption even at rest, contributing to overall metabolic health.

By understanding the potential health benefits of intermittent fasting, women over 60 can make informed decisions about incorporating this dietary approach into their lives to enhance overall well-being and longevity.

1.3 Risks of Intermittent Fasting for Women Over 60

Intermittent fasting has gained popularity as a potential strategy for weight loss and improved health in recent years. While it may offer benefits for some individuals, it's essential for women over 60 to be aware of potential risks and considerations associated with this eating pattern. As women age, their nutritional needs and hormonal balance change, which can impact how their bodies respond to fasting.

1. Hormonal Changes. Women over 60 experience significant hormonal changes, particularly related to menopause. During menopause, estrogen levels decrease, which can lead to changes in metabolism and body composition. Intermittent fasting might further impact hormonal balance, potentially leading to irregular menstrual cycles or exacerbating menopausal symptoms. It is crucial for women in this age group to pay attention to any hormonal changes and consult with a healthcare professional if they notice significant disruptions. **Recommendation:** Before starting intermittent fasting, women over 60 should discuss their health status and hormonal changes with a healthcare provider to determine if this eating pattern is suitable for them.

2. Nutrient Deficiency. As women age, their bodies may require more specific nutrients to support bone health, cognitive function, and overall well-being. Intermittent fasting can sometimes lead to reduced nutrient intake, potentially increasing the risk of deficiencies in essential vitamins and minerals. **Recommendation:** Women over 60 should focus on consuming nutrient-dense foods during their eating windows and consider supplementation if necessary. Including a variety of fruits, vegetables, whole grains, lean proteins, and healthy fats can help meet essential nutrient needs.

3. Bone Health. Postmenopausal women are at an increased risk of osteoporosis, a condition characterized by decreased bone density and increased fracture risk. Fasting can impact bone health, as it may reduce calcium intake and affect bone-building processes. **Recommendation:** To support bone health, women over 60 should ensure an adequate intake of calcium and vitamin D through dietary sources or supplements. Weight-bearing exercises should also be included in their fitness routine to promote bone strength.

4. Muscle Mass. As people age, there is a natural tendency to lose muscle mass, known as sarcopenia. Intermittent fasting, particularly when combined with inadequate protein intake, can accelerate muscle loss. **Recommendation:** Women over 60 should prioritize protein-rich foods such as lean meats, poultry, fish, dairy, legumes, and plant-based protein sources. Adequate protein intake is essential to preserve muscle mass and support overall health.

5. Blood Sugar Regulation. Intermittent fasting can impact blood sugar levels, which is particularly important for individuals with diabetes or prediabetes. Women over 60 should monitor their blood sugar levels carefully during fasting periods to avoid any adverse effects.

Recommendation: If you have diabetes or prediabetes, consult with your healthcare provider before attempting intermittent fasting. They can help tailor a fasting plan that aligns with your specific health needs and medications.

6. Hydration. Older adults, including women over 60, may have reduced thirst sensations, making them susceptible to dehydration. During fasting periods, the risk of dehydration may increase, particularly if combined with physical activity. **Recommendation:** Stay vigilant about hydration during fasting periods. Consume sufficient water and hydrating beverages to prevent dehydration and support overall health.

7. Medications and Medical Conditions. Certain medications require food intake for optimal absorption, and some medical conditions may not be compatible with fasting. Women over 60 should be cautious if they are taking medications or have underlying health conditions. **Recommendation:** Prioritize regular consultations with your healthcare provider, who can advise on adjusting medication schedules and monitor the effects of intermittent fasting on specific medical conditions.

Remember, each individual's health status, hormonal changes, and nutritional needs should be carefully considered before starting an intermittent fasting regimen. Consulting with a healthcare professional and making informed decisions about dietary choices and fasting patterns will help ensure overall well-being and safety while exploring intermittent fasting as a potential approach to health improvement.

Chapter 2: Exercise While Fasting

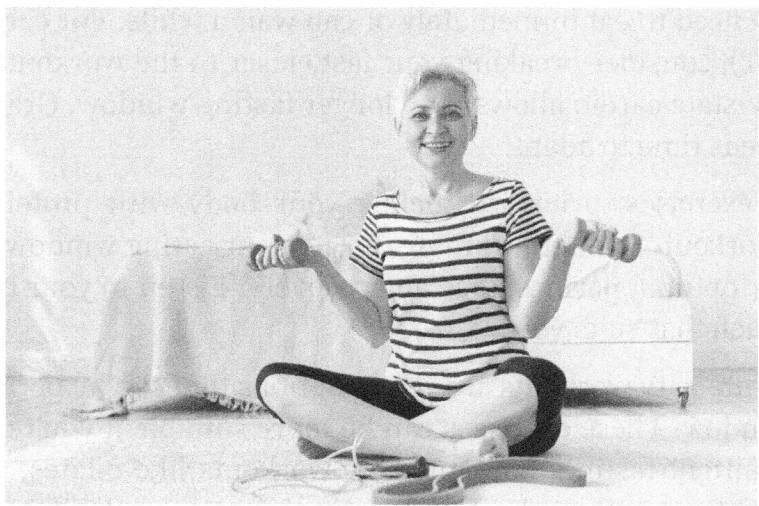

Working out while following an intermittent fasting (IF) plan may seem challenging at first. The potential feelings of weakness, fatigue, and hunger from fasting can make the idea of exercise daunting. However, many people praise the benefits of fasted cardio. So, how can you effectively and safely combine your IF plan with your workout routine?

Here is a comprehensive guide on exercising while fasting, without compromising your long-term health goals.

Can you exercise while on an intermittent fast?

In short, yes, you can exercise during fasting. However, the longer answer depends on how you feel and listen to your body. Different variations of intermittent fasting, such as the 16:8 plan or the 5:2 plan, require modifying your fasting strategy based on your workout type and the time of day you prefer to exercise. If fasting makes you too weak to work out, prioritize your nutrition first, and exercise afterward. It's essential to find a balance that works well for you, as individual preferences vary.

Benefits of working out while fasting

Exercising in a fasted state can have advantages, especially for weight loss. Research published in the Journal of Nutrition and Metabolism in 2016 showed that fasted cardio can enhance fat oxidation, meaning your body uses fat reserves as energy instead of carbohydrates from recent meals. However, whether fasted workouts suit you depends on how your body responds. Experiment with different workout schedules to find one that suits you best.

Things to look out for

While some people may feel great working out on an empty stomach, others may experience weakness or dizziness. Exercising while fasting may lead to increased fat loss but could also result in muscle loss. To prevent this, replenish your body with carbohydrates and protein, especially after a workout, to promote muscle recovery and strength.

How to choose the best exercise for your IF plan

Not all exercises are equal when it comes to intermittent fasting. The type of exercise you do may influence whether you need to eat immediately or can wait a while. For cardio and high-intensity interval training (HIIT), consider breaking your fast closer to the workout to fuel your body. On the other hand, steady-state cardio allows for a longer fasting window. Gradually ease into fasted cardio if your body needs time to adapt.

For muscle-building exercises, prioritize fueling your body with protein and complex carbs before or after your workout. Strength training during your eating window ensures your muscles have adequate fuel for optimal performance and recovery. Listen to your body's needs and goals to find the best approach that suits you.

Yoga, barre, and low-intensity workouts are gentle options that can be performed either fasted or within your eating window. These exercises can be more suitable if you're feeling low on energy or adjusting to intermittent fasting. Low-intensity workouts like pilates, yoga, or barre tend to perform better when done within the fasting window, especially if you plan on practicing intermittent fasting a few times per week.

Remember, it's essential to find a workout routine that aligns with your fasting plan and provides the best results while taking into account your body's unique needs and preferences.

2.1 14-Day Exercise Plan During Intermittent Fasting for Women Over 60

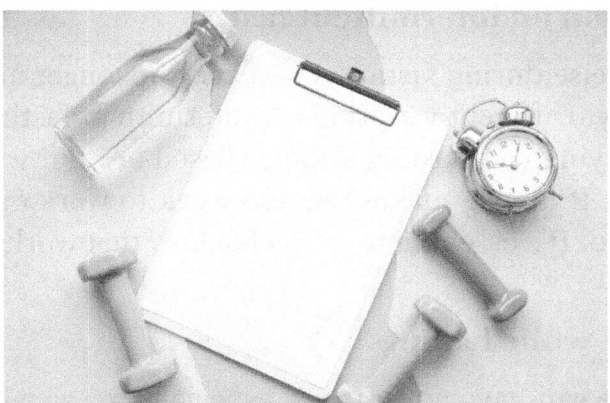

Day 1: Gentle Walk   **Duration:** 20-30 minutes

Description: Start the week with a gentle walk in your neighborhood or a nearby park. Walking is a low-impact exercise that helps improve cardiovascular health and joint flexibility.

Day 2: Chair Yoga   **Duration:** 20-30 minutes

Description: Engage in chair yoga exercises that focus on gentle stretches and breathing techniques. Chair yoga is suitable for older adults and helps improve flexibility and balance.

Day 3: Bodyweight Strength Training   Duration: 15-20 minutes

Description: Perform bodyweight exercises such as squats, modified push-ups, and seated leg lifts. These exercises help build muscle strength and support overall mobility.

Day 4: Rest Day

Description: Allow your body to recover and rest on this day. Practice light stretching or relaxation exercises.

Day 5: Water Aerobics or Swimming   Duration: 20-30 minutes

Description: If possible, engage in water aerobics or swimming. Water exercises are gentle on joints and provide resistance for muscle toning.

Day 6: Balance Exercises   Duration: 15-20 minutes

Description: Practice balance exercises like standing on one leg or heel-to-toe walking. Balance exercises help reduce the risk of falls and improve stability.

Day 7: Rest Day

Description: Take another rest day to allow your body to recover and rejuvenate.

Day 8: Low-impact Cardio   Duration: 20-30 minutes

Description: Engage in low-impact cardio exercises such as stationary biking or using an elliptical machine. These exercises elevate your heart rate without putting stress on your joints.

Day 9: Resistance Band Workout   Duration: 15-20 minutes

Description: Use resistance bands to perform exercises like bicep curls, shoulder presses, and leg lifts. Resistance bands offer a safe and effective way to strengthen muscles.

Day 10: Restorative Yoga   Duration: 20-30 minutes

Description: Practice restorative yoga poses that focus on deep relaxation and stress relief. Restorative yoga is gentle and promotes a sense of calmness.

Day 11: Light Dance Workout   Duration: 15-20 minutes

Description: Put on your favorite music and do some light dancing. Dancing is a fun way to stay active and improve coordination.

Day 12: Stretching and Flexibility   **Duration:** 15-20 minutes

Description: Spend time on stretching exercises to improve flexibility and reduce muscle tension.

Day 13: Tai Chi   **Duration:** 20-30 minutes

Description: Try Tai Chi, a slow and gentle martial art that focuses on balance and mindfulness. Tai Chi is excellent for improving body awareness and relaxation.

Day 14: Mindful Walking   **Duration:** 20-30 minutes

Description: End the plan with a mindful walk, focusing on your breath and surroundings. Mindful walking promotes mental clarity and emotional well-being.

Remember to stay hydrated and listen to your body throughout the plan. If any exercise feels too strenuous or causes discomfort, modify it or consult with a fitness professional. Always start with a warm-up and end with a cool-down session to prevent injuries.

2.2 Tips for Working Out While Intermittent Fasting

Remember to stay hydrated and listen to your body throughout the plan. If any exercise feels too strenuous or causes discomfort, modify it or consult with a fitness professional. Always start with a warm-up and end with a cool-down session to prevent injuries.

Ease into it: As you start working out while intermittent fasting, gradually increase the intensity and duration of your workouts to allow your body to adjust to the new eating regimen. Begin with shorter, low-intensity exercises and gradually work your way up to longer sessions.

Consider the timing: Choose the best time of day for your workouts based on your eating schedule and personal preferences. If you exercise in the morning, plan to eat after a cardio session, and if you prefer late afternoons, focus on weight training. Low-intensity workouts can be done at any time of day.

Be flexible with your eating window: Adjust your eating schedule to fit in with your workout routine. If you like morning runs, consider shifting your eating window to accommodate a post-workout protein shake.

Stay hydrated: Don't forget to drink plenty of water, especially when exercising while fasting. Aim for at least 72 ounces of water daily to stay hydrated, especially if you sweat a lot during workouts.

Use electrolytes: Incorporate natural sports drinks or low-calorie options like coconut water to replenish electrolytes without breaking your fast.

Mix up your workouts: Combine both strength training and cardio exercises to promote fat burning and muscle development. Adapt your workout focus depending on the time of day you exercise.

Listen to your body: Pay attention to how you feel during and after workouts. Choose exercises that leave you feeling energized and strong rather than exhausted. Avoid overexerting yourself and be mindful of signs of fatigue or strain.

Alternate-day fasting: On days with significant calorie restriction, opt for low-intensity or no workouts. Avoid pushing your body to extreme exertion on fasting days to prevent depletion and potential injury.

Experiment and find what works for you: Each individual may respond differently to intermittent fasting and exercise combinations. Try out various workout routines and schedules to discover what suits you best.

Remember the purpose of intermittent fasting: Intermittent fasting is about eating on a schedule, not skipping meals. Ensure that you consume your daily calories and essential nutrients within the designated eating window for optimal results.

2.3 Yoga and Intermittent Fasting: Combining for Optimal Health

Yoga practitioners often prioritize their health and well-being, and weight management is a significant aspect of this journey. As a result, many yoga enthusiasts wonder if intermittent fasting is suitable for their practice. When done correctly, intermittent fasting can be integrated into a yoga routine, but certain precautions should be taken, especially for pregnant women or those with specific health conditions.

Understanding Yoga

Yoga encompasses various disciplines and practices that originated in India but have evolved into physical exercises, relaxation techniques, and stress relief practices. Different styles of yoga are prevalent in the West, with some focusing on physical postures (hatha) and others emphasizing mental and spiritual aspects (mantra, laya). It aims to holistically benefit the mind, body, and spirit, combining postures (asanas), meditation, and controlled breathing (ujjayi or pranayama) to create a harmonious session.

The Benefits of Yoga

Yoga offers a wide range of benefits, including:

- Weight loss
- Reduced inflammation
- Stress and anxiety relief
- Improved heart health
- Enhanced flexibility and balance
- Increased cognitive function

- Alleviated depression
- Improved breathing and chronic pain relief
- Promotion of healthy eating habits
- Enhanced quality of life

Weight Loss Effectiveness

Yoga can contribute to weight loss and weight management through various mechanisms. Dynamic and flowing yoga styles, such as Ashtanga, Bikram, Iyengar, and Kundalini, can provide excellent aerobic exercise and calorie burning. Additionally, mindfulness, a fundamental aspect of yoga, helps practitioners make healthier food choices and develop better eating habits, supporting weight loss efforts.

Best Yoga Practice Times During Intermittent Fasting

The timing of yoga practice during intermittent fasting can be a concern. To optimize benefits and ensure safety, it is advisable to practice yoga before or just after the fasting hours. This way, your body will have enough energy reserves to sustain your yoga session. Exercising or doing yoga on an empty stomach can enhance weight loss as the body taps into fat stores for energy, a process known as metabolic switching.

Stress Relief Effectiveness

Yoga is renowned for its stress-reducing properties. Even physically demanding styles like Ashtanga and hot yoga can help alleviate stress, anxiety, and depression. Yoga's ability to reduce cortisol levels, the stress hormone, contributes to its stress-relief benefits.

Intermittent Fasting and Stress:

Intermittent fasting can temporarily increase cortisol levels, similar to exercise. However, yoga's stress-reducing effects can counteract any negative impact from fasting. Staying well-hydrated throughout the day can also help mitigate stress effects during fasting.

Combining Yoga and Intermittent Fasting:

When combined thoughtfully, yoga and intermittent fasting can complement each other for optimal health. While intermittent fasting alone may not be the best stress-reduction strategy, incorporating yoga into your routine can counteract any negative effects. As your body adjusts to the new routine and you begin to experience weight loss benefits, the journey becomes more manageable and rewarding.

Yoga and intermittent fasting can work together harmoniously, promoting overall well-being. Mindfulness from yoga can support healthy eating habits during fasting, and yoga's stress-relief benefits can counteract any stress induced by intermittent fasting. As with any lifestyle change, listen to your body, and adjust your practices accordingly for a personalized and fulfilling journey toward optimal health and wellness.

Chapter 3: Breakfast Recipes For Intermittent Fasting

1. Poached Eggs & Avocado Toasts

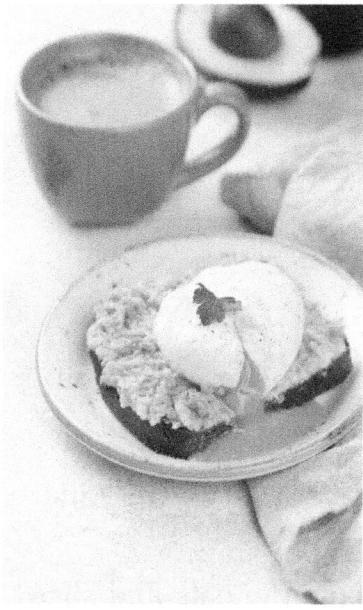

(Ready in: 15 minutes | Serves: 4)

Ingredients:

- 2 ripe avocados
- 4 eggs
- 2 teaspoons lemon juice (or juice of 1 lime)
- 1 cup cheese (grated, edam, gruyere, or whatever you have on hand)
- 4 slices thick bread
- 4 teaspoons butter (for spreading on toast)
- Salt & freshly ground black pepper

Instructions:

- Poach the eggs using your favorite technique. Cut the avocados in half and remove the stones. Scoop out the flesh into a bowl with a spoon. Add the lemon or lime juice, salt, and pepper, and mash using a fork.

- Toast the bread and spread with butter. Spread the avocado mixture on each slice of buttered toast and top each one with a poached egg.

- Sprinkle the grated cheese over the eggs and serve immediately. These are also delicious with tomato halves on the side, either fresh or grilled.

Nutritional Info: Calories: 421 kcal, Protein: 18g, Carbohydrates: 25g, Fat: 28g

2. French Vanilla Almond Granola

(Ready in: 2 hrs 10 mins | Serves: 12 | Yield: 12 1/2 cup servings)

Ingredients:

- 1/2 cup sliced almonds
- 3 1/2 cups old-fashioned oats
- 1/2 cup water
- 1/4 teaspoon salt
- 1/2 cup natural cane sugar
- 1 tablespoon vanilla extract
- 1/4 cup organic canola oil or 1/4 cup grapeseed oil

Instructions:

- Preheat the oven to 200°F (93°C). Line a large, rimmed cookie sheet with parchment paper.
- In a large bowl, combine the oats and sliced almonds. In a small saucepan over medium heat, stir the water, sugar, and salt until the sugar is dissolved. Remove from heat and stir in the vanilla extract and canola oil.
- Pour the sugar-oil mixture over the oat-almond mixture and stir until well coated. Spread the mixture on the lined cookie sheet and bake for 2 hours, or until the granola is tender to the touch. Do not stir during baking.
- Remove from the oven and allow to cool into chunks before breaking apart. Store in an airtight container.

Nutritional Info: Calories: 190 kcal, Protein: 3g, Carbohydrates: 21g, Fat: 11g

3. Baked Potato

(Ready in: 1hr 10mins | Serves: 1)

Ingredients:

- Canola oil
- One large russet potato
- Kosher salt

Instructions:

- Preheat the oven to 350°F (175°C) and position the racks in the upper and lower thirds of the oven.

- Thoroughly wash the potato with a stiff brush and cold running water. Pat it dry and use a regular fork to poke 8 to 12 deep holes all over the potato, allowing moisture to escape during cooking.
- Place the potato in a bowl and gently coat it with canola oil. Sprinkle kosher salt evenly over the potato's surface.
- Place the potato directly on the middle rack of the oven. To catch any drippings, place a baking sheet or a piece of aluminum foil on the lower rack.
- Bake the potato for about 1 hour or until the skin feels crisp and the flesh feels soft underneath.
- To serve, create a dotted line with your fork from end to end of the potato, then gently crack it open by pressing the ends towards each other. The potato should pop open, revealing its fluffy interior.

Nutritional Info: Calories: 278 kcal, Protein: 6g, Carbohydrates: 63g, Fat: 1g, Fiber: 7g, Sodium: 21mg

5. Vegan Coconut Kefir Banana Muffins

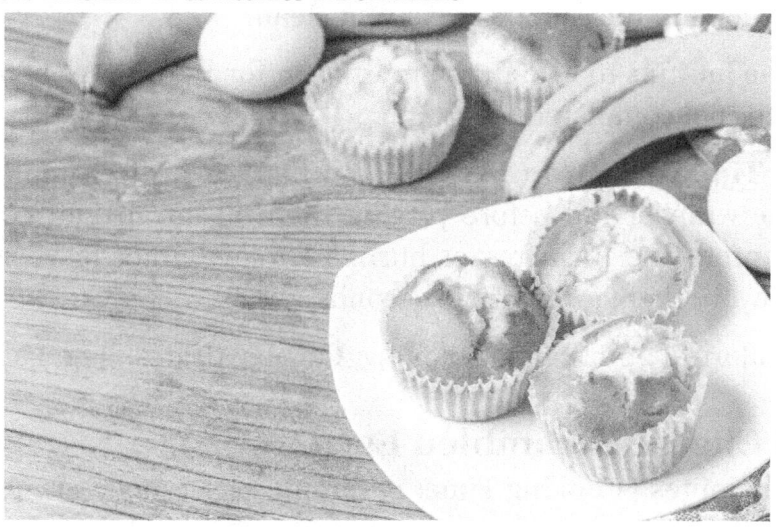

(Preparation Time: 45 minutes | Servings: 12)

Ingredients:

- 2 cups all-purpose flour
- 1 cup unsweetened dried shredded coconut
- 1 cup granulated sugar
- 2 teaspoons baking soda
- 1/2 teaspoon salt
- 2 ripe bananas, mashed
- 1 teaspoon baking powder

- 1/4 cup cold-pressed liquid coconut oil
- 1 1/2 cups dairy-free kefir probiotic fermented coconut milk
- 1 teaspoon vanilla extract

Instructions:

- Preheat the oven to 180°C (350°F) and lightly grease a 12-count muffin tin or line it with muffin liners.
- In a large bowl, whisk together the flour, sugar, dried coconut, baking soda, baking powder, and salt.
- In a separate large bowl, whisk together the mashed bananas, kefir, coconut oil, and vanilla.
- Combine the wet ingredients with the dry ingredients and stir until there are no white streaks left.
- Divide the muffin batter evenly between the prepared muffin tin wells.
- Bake in the preheated oven for about 30 minutes or until the tops are golden and a toothpick inserted into the centers comes out clean.
- Allow the muffins to cool in the muffin tin for 15 minutes before transferring them to a wire rack to cool completely.
- **Chef's Tip:** You can freeze these muffins for up to a month. Individually wrap them in plastic wrap or foil before placing them in an airtight container or resealable freezer bag to protect against freezer burn. To thaw, either leave them overnight in the fridge or microwave them for 20 to 30 seconds.

Nutritional Info: Calories: 260 kcal, Protein: 3g, Carbohydrates: 32g, Fat: 13g

6. Zucchini and Cheese Scrambled Eggs

(Preparation Time: 4 minutes | Cooking Time: 15 minutes | Servings: 1)

Ingredients:

- 1 small yellow onion, thinly sliced (about 4 ounces)
- 1 1/2 tablespoons olive oil, divided
- 2-3 garlic cloves, sliced in half
- 1 small zucchini, chopped into ½-inch quarters (about 6 ounces)
- 1 egg, at room temperature, slightly beaten
- Salt and pepper, to taste
- 1 tablespoon water
- 1 tablespoon chopped Italian parsley

- 1-2 tablespoons grated Romano cheese

Instructions:

- In a large skillet, heat 1 tablespoon of olive oil over medium-high heat. Add the sliced onion and reduce the heat to medium. Cook, stirring occasionally, until the onion becomes translucent and softened, about 3-5 minutes.

- Add the remaining chopped zucchini, 1/2 tablespoon of olive oil, and the sliced garlic to the skillet. Season with salt and pepper.

- Saute the zucchini, stirring and shaking the pan, until it turns golden brown and is cooked but still crisp, about 7-10 minutes. Adjust the heat as needed. Whisk together the grated Romano cheese and chopped parsley with the beaten egg.

- Once the zucchini is cooked, pour the egg mixture into the skillet and let it cook for about 30 seconds. Stir and shake the pan until the egg is scrambled and set, which should take about 1 minute.

- Taste and adjust the seasonings if necessary. Serve immediately, garnishing with additional chopped Italian parsley and grated Romano cheese if desired.

Nutritional Info: Calories: 280kcal, Carbohydrates: 17g, Protein: 10g, Fat: 20g, Saturated Fat: 4g, Sodium: 141mg, Potassium: 529mg, Cholesterol: 169mg, Fiber: 3g, Sugar: 8g, Iron: 2mg, Vitamin A: 811IU, Vitamin C: 36mg, Calcium: 133mg

7. Egg Scramble with Sweet Potatoes

(Preparation Time: 10 minutes | Cooking Time: 20 minutes | Servings: 2)

Ingredients:

- 1/2 cup chopped onion
- 1 (8-oz) sweet potato, diced
- 2 teaspoons chopped rosemary
- Salt, to taste
- 4 large eggs
- 4 large egg whites
- Pepper, to taste
- 2 tablespoons chopped chives

Instructions:

- Preheat the oven to 425°F (220°C). On a baking dish, toss the diced sweet potato, chopped onion, chopped rosemary, salt, and pepper. Spray with cooking spray and roast for about 20 minutes, or until the sweet potatoes are tender.

- In a medium bowl, whisk together the eggs, egg whites, and a pinch of salt and pepper. Spray a skillet with cooking spray and scramble the eggs over medium heat for about 5 minutes.
- Serve the scrambled eggs with the roasted sweet potatoes and sprinkle with chopped chives.

Nutritional Info: Calories: 571, Protein: 44g, Carbohydrates: 52g (including 9g of fiber). Fat: 20g

8. Spicy Spanish Tomato Baked Eggs

(Cooking Time: 15 minutes | Servings: 2)

Ingredients:

- 1 tablespoon olive oil
- 1 red pepper, deseeded and cut into strips
- 2 red onions, peeled and cut into half-moons
- 1 clove garlic, peeled and sliced
- 1 teaspoon paprika
- 4 medium eggs
- 250g cherry tomatoes, halved (or 1 tin peeled plum tomatoes)
- 2 tablespoons chopped flat-leaf parsley (optional)

Instructions:

- Preheat the oven to 180°C (350°F). In a large, deep, ovenproof frying pan, heat the olive oil. Add the onions, garlic, and red pepper. Season with freshly ground black pepper and cook over medium heat until soft, about 10 minutes. Add the tomatoes and paprika, and cook gently for an additional 5 minutes.
- Create four small wells in the tomato mixture and crack an egg into each. Season with salt and pepper, then cover the pan and place it in the oven.
- Bake until the eggs are set, about 5-8 minutes. If desired, sprinkle chopped flat-leaf parsley on top before serving.

Nutritional Info: Calories: 250, Protein: 12g, Carbohydrates: 18g, Fat: 15g, Fiber: 4g

9. Smoked Salmon and Avocado Wrap

(Prep Time: 10 minutes | Servings: 2)

Ingredients:

- 4 large lettuce leaves (such as romaine or butter lettuce)
- 4 ounces smoked salmon

- 1 ripe avocado, sliced
- 1/4 red onion, thinly sliced
- 1 tablespoon capers
- 2 teaspoons lemon juice
- Salt and pepper to taste

Instructions:
- Lay out the lettuce leaves on a clean surface.
- Divide the smoked salmon, avocado slices, and red onion evenly among the lettuce leaves. Sprinkle capers over the filling and drizzle with lemon juice.
- Season with salt and pepper to taste. Carefully roll up the lettuce leaves to form wraps. Serve immediately or wrap in parchment paper for a portable breakfast.

Nutritional Info: Calories: 190kcal | Carbohydrates: 6g | Protein: 13g | Fat: 13g | Saturated Fat: 2g | Cholesterol: 16mg | Sodium: 537mg | Fiber: 4g | Sugar: 1g | Vitamin A: 1429IU | Vitamin C: 11mg | Calcium: 25mg | Iron: 1mg

10. Almond Flour Pancakes with Sugar-Free Syrup

(Prep Time: 5 minutes | Cook Time: 10 minutes | Servings: 2)

Ingredients:
- 1 cup almond flour
- 2 large eggs
- 1/4 cup unsweetened almond milk
- 1 tablespoon melted butter
- 1 teaspoon baking powder
- 1/2 teaspoon vanilla extract
- Pinch of salt
- Sugar-free pancake syrup (for serving)

Instructions:
- In a mixing bowl, whisk together almond flour, eggs, almond milk, melted butter, baking powder, vanilla extract, and salt until smooth. Heat a non-stick skillet over medium heat and lightly grease it with cooking spray or butter.
- Pour about 1/4 cup of the pancake batter onto the skillet to form each pancake. Cook until bubbles form on the surface, then flip and cook until golden brown on both sides. Repeat with the remaining batter to make additional pancakes.
- Serve the pancakes with sugar-free syrup.

Nutritional Info: Calories: 370kcal | Carbohydrates: 10g | Protein: 16g | Fat: 31g | Saturated Fat: 7g | Cholesterol: 186mg | Sodium: 444mg | Fiber: 5g | Sugar: 1g | Vitamin A: 469IU | Calcium: 250mg | Iron: 3mg

11. Green Smoothie with Spinach, Kale, and Pineapple

(Prep Time: 5 minutes | Servings: 2)

Ingredients:

- 1 cup fresh spinach leaves
- 1 cup fresh kale leaves
- 1 cup frozen pineapple chunks
- 1 ripe banana
- 1 cup unsweetened almond milk
- 1 tablespoon chia seeds (optional)
- Ice cubes (optional)

Instructions:

- In a blender, combine spinach, kale, frozen pineapple, banana, and almond milk. Blend until smooth and creamy. Add chia seeds if desired and blend for a few more seconds. If you prefer a colder smoothie, add a few ice cubes and blend again. Pour the smoothie into glasses and serve immediately.

Nutritional Info: Calories: 160kcal | Carbohydrates: 31g | Protein: 4g | Fat: 4g | Saturated Fat: 1g | Cholesterol: 0mg | Sodium: 160mg | Fiber: 5g | Sugar: 17g | Vitamin A: 4879IU | Vitamin C: 64mg | Calcium: 258mg | Iron: 2mg

12. Chia Seed Pudding with Mixed Berries

(Prep Time: 5 minutes | Refrigeration time: 4 hours or overnight|Servings: 2)

Ingredients:

- 1/4 cup chia seeds
- 1 cup unsweetened almond milk
- 1 tablespoon honey or maple syrup
- 1/2 teaspoon vanilla extract
- Mixed berries (such as strawberries, blueberries, and raspberries) for topping

Instructions:

- In a bowl, whisk together chia seeds, almond milk, honey (or maple syrup), and vanilla extract until well combined.

- Cover the bowl and refrigerate for at least 4 hours or overnight, allowing the chia seeds to absorb the liquid and thicken.
- Before serving, give the pudding a good stir to ensure it's evenly thickened.
- Top with mixed berries and serve chilled.

Nutritional Info: Calories: 180kcal | Carbohydrates: 21g | Protein: 5g | Fat: 8g | Saturated Fat: 1g | Cholesterol: 0mg | Sodium: 85mg | Fiber: 10g | Sugar: 8g | Vitamin A: 55IU | Vitamin C: 0.2mg | Calcium: 320mg | Iron: 2.7mg

13. Quinoa Breakfast Bowl with Nuts and Seeds

(Prep Time: 5 minutes | Cook Time: 15 minutes | Servings: 2)

Ingredients:

- 1/2 cup quinoa, rinsed
- 1 cup water
- 1/2 cup Greek yogurt
- 2 tablespoons chopped nuts (such as almonds, walnuts, or pistachios)
- 1 tablespoon mixed seeds (such as chia seeds, flaxseeds, or pumpkin seeds)
- 1 tablespoon honey or maple syrup
- 1/2 cup fresh berries (such as blueberries, strawberries, or raspberries)
- A pinch of cinnamon (optional)

Instructions:

- In a small saucepan, combine quinoa and water. Bring to a boil, then reduce heat to low and simmer for about 15 minutes or until the quinoa is cooked and water is absorbed. Fluff the quinoa with a fork.
- Divide the cooked quinoa into two serving bowls.
- Top each bowl with Greek yogurt, chopped nuts, mixed seeds, and fresh berries.
- Drizzle honey or maple syrup over the toppings.
- Sprinkle a pinch of cinnamon on top if desired. Serve immediately and enjoy!

Nutritional Info: Calories: 315kcal | Carbohydrates: 42g | Protein: 13g | Fat: 11g | Saturated Fat: 2g | Cholesterol: 5mg | Sodium: 25mg | Fiber: 6g | Sugar: 14g | Vitamin A: 68IU | Vitamin C: 8mg | Calcium: 138mg | Iron: 3mg

14. Low-Carb Vegetable Omelette

(Prep Time: 10 minutes | Cook Time: 10 minutes | Servings: 2)

Ingredients:

- 3 large eggs
- 1 tablespoon milk (or unsweetened almond milk)
- Salt and pepper to taste
- 1/2 cup chopped mixed vegetables (such as bell peppers, spinach, tomatoes, onions, or mushrooms)
- 1 tablespoon grated cheese (such as cheddar or feta)
- 1 teaspoon olive oil

Instructions:

- In a bowl, whisk together eggs, milk, salt, and pepper until well combined.
- Heat olive oil in a non-stick skillet over medium heat.
- Add the chopped vegetables to the skillet and sauté until they are tender, about 3-4 minutes.
- Pour the egg mixture over the vegetables in the skillet. Cook the omelette for about 3 minutes, or until the edges start to set.
- Sprinkle grated cheese over half of the omelette.
- Carefully fold the omelette in half using a spatula.
- Cook for another 2 minutes, or until the cheese is melted and the omelette is fully cooked. Slide the omelette onto a plate and serve hot.

Nutritional Info: Calories: 325kcal | Carbohydrates: 8g | Protein: 22g | Fat: 23g | Saturated Fat: 8g | Cholesterol: 498mg | Sodium: 356mg | Fiber: 2g | Sugar: 4g | Vitamin A: 3545IU | Vitamin C: 49mg | Calcium: 196mg | Iron: 3mg

15. Greek Yogurt Parfait with Berries and Almonds

(Prep Time: 5 minutes | Servings: 1)

Ingredients:

- 1 cup Greek yogurt
- 1/2 cup mixed berries (such as strawberries, blueberries, and raspberries)
- 2 tablespoons sliced almonds
- 1 tablespoon honey or maple syrup
- A pinch of cinnamon (optional)

Instructions:

- In a serving glass or bowl, layer half of the Greek yogurt.
- Add half of the mixed berries on top of the yogurt.
- Sprinkle half of the sliced almonds over the berries.
- Drizzle half of the honey or maple syrup over the almonds.
- Repeat the layers with the remaining ingredients.
- If desired, sprinkle a pinch of cinnamon on top. Serve immediately and enjoy!

Nutritional Info: Calories: 340kcal | Carbohydrates: 31g | Protein: 18g | Fat: 17g | Saturated Fat: 3g | Cholesterol: 16mg | Sodium: 59mg | Fiber: 5g | Sugar: 21g | Vitamin A: 108IU | Vitamin C: 5mg | Calcium: 280mg | Iron: 2mg

16. Cinnamon Walnut Baked Apples

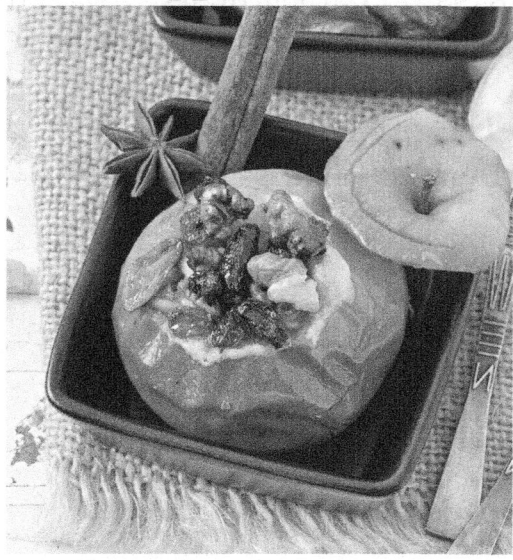

(Prep Time: 10 minutes | Cook Time: 30 minutes | Servings: 4)

Ingredients:

- 4 medium-sized apples (such as Granny Smith or Honeycrisp)
- 1/4 cup chopped walnuts
- 2 tablespoons honey or maple syrup
- 1 teaspoon ground cinnamon
- 1/4 teaspoon ground nutmeg
- 1 tablespoon melted butter or coconut oil
- 1/2 cup water

Instructions:

- Preheat the oven to 375°F (190°C). Core the apples to remove the seeds, leaving the bottom intact.
- In a small bowl, mix together the chopped walnuts, honey or maple syrup, ground cinnamon, ground nutmeg, and melted butter or coconut oil.
- Stuff each apple with the walnut mixture and place them in a baking dish. Pour the water into the bottom of the baking dish to create steam while baking.
- Cover the baking dish with aluminum foil and bake in the preheated oven for 20 minutes.
- Remove the foil and bake for an additional 10 minutes, or until the apples are tender and slightly caramelized.
- Serve warm, optionally with a dollop of Greek yogurt or a sprinkle of additional cinnamon on top.

Nutritional Info: Calories: 185 kcal | Carbohydrates: 30g | Protein: 2g | Fat: 8g | Saturated Fat: 2g | Sodium: 3mg | Fiber: 5g | Sugar: 21g | Vitamin C: 8mg | Calcium: 28mg | Iron: 1mg

17. Zucchini and Spinach Egg Muffins

(Prep Time: 10 minutes | Cook Time: 20 minutes | Servings: 6)

Ingredients:

- 6 large eggs
- 1 cup chopped zucchini
- 1 cup chopped spinach
- 1/2 cup diced red bell pepper
- 1/4 cup chopped green onions
- 1/4 cup grated Parmesan cheese
- 1/2 teaspoon garlic powder
- 1/2 teaspoon dried oregano
- Salt and pepper to taste
- Cooking spray

Instructions:

- Preheat the oven to 375°F (190°C). Grease a muffin tin with cooking spray. In a large bowl, whisk the eggs. Add the chopped zucchini, spinach, red bell pepper, green onions, Parmesan cheese, garlic powder, dried oregano, salt, and pepper.
- Mix well to combine. Pour the egg mixture into the prepared muffin tin, filling each cup about 3/4 full.

- Bake in the preheated oven for 15-20 minutes, or until the egg muffins are set and slightly golden on top. Remove from the oven and let them cool slightly before serving.

Nutritional Info: Calories: 96 kcal | Carbohydrates: 3g | Protein: 8g | Fat: 6g | Saturated Fat: 2g | Cholesterol: 186mg | Sodium: 135mg | Fiber: 1g | Sugar: 1g | Vitamin A: 1123IU | Vitamin C: 13mg | Calcium: 73mg | Iron: 1mg

18. Broccoli and Cheddar Mini Crustless Quiches

(Prep Time: 15 minutes | Cook Time: 25 minutes | Servings: 6)

Ingredients:

- 6 large eggs
- 1 cup chopped broccoli florets
- 1/2 cup shredded cheddar cheese
- 1/4 cup chopped red onion
- 1/4 cup milk (or non-dairy milk)
- 1/2 teaspoon garlic powder
- Salt and pepper to taste
- Cooking spray

Instructions:

- Preheat the oven to 375°F (190°C). Grease a muffin tin with cooking spray. In a large bowl, whisk the eggs. Add the chopped broccoli, shredded cheddar cheese, chopped red onion, milk, garlic powder, salt, and pepper. Mix well to combine. Pour the egg mixture into the prepared muffin tin, filling each cup about 3/4 full.
- Bake in the preheated oven for 20-25 minutes, or until the mini quiches are set and slightly golden on top. Remove from the oven and let them cool slightly before serving.

Nutritional Info: Calories: 118 kcal | Carbohydrates: 2g | Protein: 8g | Fat: 8g | Saturated Fat: 4g | Cholesterol: 184mg | Sodium: 166mg | Fiber: 1g | Sugar: 1g | Vitamin A: 586IU | Vitamin C: 16mg | Calcium: 117mg | Iron: 1mg

19. Blueberry Protein Smoothie

(Prep Time: 5 minutes | Servings: 1)

Ingredients:

- 1 cup unsweetened almond milk (or any non-dairy milk)
- 1/2 cup frozen blueberries
- 1/2 banana
- 1 tablespoon almond butter

- 1 tablespoon chia seeds
- 1 scoop vanilla protein powder (plant-based or whey)
- Optional: honey or maple syrup to sweeten, if desired

Instructions:

- In a blender, combine the unsweetened almond milk, frozen blueberries, banana, almond butter, chia seeds, and vanilla protein powder. Blend until smooth and creamy. If desired, add honey or maple syrup to sweeten the smoothie to your taste. Pour the smoothie into a glass and enjoy immediately.

Nutritional Info: Calories: 326 kcal | Carbohydrates: 30g | Protein: 25g | Fat: 14g | Saturated Fat: 2g | Sodium: 351mg | Fiber: 11g | Sugar: 14g | Vitamin C: 17mg | Calcium: 501mg | Iron: 4mg

20. Vegetable Frittata with Turmeric and Herbs

(Prep Time: 10 minutes | Cook Time: 20 minutes | Servings: 4)

Ingredients:

- 6 large eggs
- 1/2 cup chopped red bell pepper
- 1/2 cup chopped zucchini
- 1/2 cup chopped spinach
- 1/4 cup chopped fresh herbs (such as parsley, chives, or basil)
- 1 teaspoon ground turmeric
- Salt and pepper to taste
- 1 tablespoon olive oil

Instructions:

- Preheat the oven to 375°F (190°C). In a large bowl, whisk the eggs. Add the chopped red bell pepper, zucchini, spinach, chopped fresh herbs, ground turmeric, salt, and pepper. Mix well to combine. Heat the olive oil in an oven-safe skillet over medium heat. Pour the egg mixture into the skillet.

- Cook the frittata on the stovetop for 2-3 minutes, or until the edges start to set. Transfer the skillet to the preheated oven and bake for 15-18 minutes, or until the frittata is fully set and slightly golden on top. Remove from the oven and let it cool slightly before slicing and serving.

Nutritional Info: Calories: 160 kcal | Carbohydrates: 4g | Protein: 11g | Fat: 11g | Saturated Fat: 3g | Cholesterol: 279mg | Sodium: 137mg | Fiber: 1g | Sugar: 2g | Vitamin A: 1984IU | Vitamin C: 23mg | Calcium: 53mg | Iron: 2mg

Chapter 4: Lunch Recipes For Intermittent Fasting

1. Baked Mahi Mahi

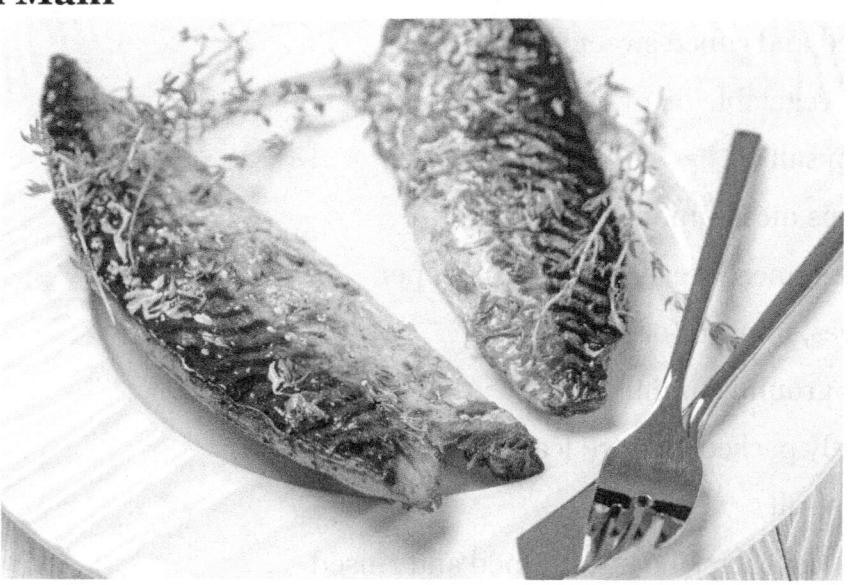

(Ready in: 40 mins | Serves: 4)

Ingredients:

- 2 lbs mahi-mahi (4 fillets)
- ¼ teaspoon garlic powder
- Juice of one lemon
- 1 cup mayonnaise
- ¼ cup finely chopped white onion
- ¼ teaspoon ground black pepper
- Breadcrumbs (optional)

Instructions:

1. Preheat the oven to 425 degrees Fahrenheit (220°C).
2. Rinse the mahi-mahi fillets and pat them dry with paper towels. Place them in a baking dish. Squeeze lemon juice over the fish and sprinkle with garlic powder, salt, and black pepper. In a small bowl, mix mayonnaise and finely chopped onion. Spread the mixture over the fish fillets.
3. Optionally, sprinkle breadcrumbs on top for added texture and flavor. Bake in the preheated oven for 25 minutes or until the fish is cooked through and flakes easily with a fork. Serve the baked Mahi Mahi with your favorite side dishes or a fresh salad.

Nutritional Info: Calories: 240 kcal, Protein: 10 g, Carbohydrates: 4 g, Fat: 19 g

2. Sweet Potato and Black Bean Burrito

(Ready in: 1hr, 5mins | Serves: 1 burrito)

Ingredients:

- 2 cups peeled and cubed sweet potatoes
- 2 teaspoons vegetable oil or vegetable broth
- 1/2 teaspoon salt
- 1 and 1/2 cups diced onions
- 1 tablespoon minced fresh green chili pepper
- 4 garlic cloves, minced (or pressed)
- 4 teaspoons ground cumin
- 1/2 cup lightly packed cilantro leaves
- 1/2 teaspoon salt
- 1 can (15 ounces) black beans, drained and rinsed
- 1 teaspoon ground coriander
- 2 tablespoons fresh lemon juice
- 12 (10 inches) flour tortillas
- Fresh salsa for topping

Instructions:

1. Preheat the oven to 350°F (175°C).

2. In a medium saucepan, add the cubed sweet potatoes and enough water to cover them. Add 1/2 teaspoon of salt. Bring to a boil, then reduce the heat to a simmer and cook for about 10 minutes until the sweet potatoes are tender. Drain and set aside.

3. In a medium saucepan or skillet, heat the vegetable oil or vegetable broth over medium-low heat. Add the diced onions, minced garlic, and green chili pepper. Cover and cook, stirring occasionally, until the onions are tender (about 7 minutes).

4. Add the ground cumin and ground coriander to the onion mixture. Cook, stirring constantly, for an additional 2 to 3 minutes. Remove from heat and set aside.

5. In a food processor, combine the cooked sweet potatoes, black beans, fresh lemon juice, cilantro leaves, and 1/2 teaspoon of salt. Blend until smooth, or mash the ingredients together in a large bowl by hand.

6. Transfer the sweet potato and black bean mixture to the large mixing bowl and mix in the cooked onion and spice mixture.

7. Lightly oil a large baking dish. Spoon about 2/3 to 3/4 cup of the filling into the center of each tortilla. Roll up the tortillas and place them seam side down in the baking dish. Cover the baking dish with foil and bake for 30 minutes, or until the burritos are heated through. Serve the Sweet Potato and Black Bean Burritos with fresh salsa on top.

Nutritional Info: Calories: 353 kcal, Protein: 8g, Carbohydrates: 59g, Fat: 9g, Fiber: 10g, Sugar: 4g, Sodium: 654mg

3. Warm Roasted Vegetable Farro Salad

(Preparation Time: 30 minutes | Cooking Time: 1 hour | Serves: 4)

Ingredients:

- 1 tablespoon kosher salt or sea salt
- 1/2 medium-sized eggplant, peel on, and large diced
- 1 cup cherry tomatoes, washed and left whole
- 6 white button mushrooms, quartered
- 1 medium-sized zucchini, peel on, and large diced
- 6 garlic cloves, peeled, trimmed, and sliced
- 1/2 medium-sized red onion, peeled and cut into wedges
- 1 cup cracked farro
- 2 cups almond milk (Almond Breeze)
- 1 tablespoon olive oil
- 1 teaspoon olive oil (15 mL)
- 1 tablespoon balsamic vinegar
- 3 sprigs fresh cilantro
- 1/2 teaspoon salt
- 1/2 teaspoon pepper
- Fresh lemon (for garnish)

Instructions:

- Preheat the oven to 200°C (400°F). Sprinkle kosher salt or sea salt over the diced eggplant in a wide flat pan or baking sheet.
- Toss the eggplant to ensure even coating, and let it sit for 30 minutes to release excess moisture and bitterness. After 30 minutes, drain the eggplant and rinse it. Transfer the eggplant to a large mixing bowl.
- Add cherry tomatoes, zucchini, mushrooms, garlic, and red onion to the bowl with the eggplant. Generously drizzle olive oil over the vegetables and season with salt and pepper. Stir to coat the vegetables evenly.

- Line an ovenproof pan with tin foil and transfer the seasoned vegetables to it. Roast the vegetables in the preheated oven for 20-25 minutes or until they become tender, caramelized, and fork-tender. Stir or flip the vegetables about halfway through the roasting process to prevent sticking.
- While the vegetables are roasting, rinse the farro under water and drain it in a colander. In a 3-quart (3L) saucepot, add the farro and almond milk. Season with a pinch of salt and drizzle with olive oil. Bring the liquid to a boil over medium-high heat, then reduce the heat to a gentle simmer. Cover the pot with a slightly ajar lid and simmer the farro for 20 minutes to release steam. Afterward, turn off the heat but leave the pot covered for another 5 minutes, allowing the farro to become soft yet slightly chewy in the middle.
- Fluff the farro with a fork. Once the vegetables are done roasting and the farro is cooked, combine them in a large serving dish. Gently toss to mix until all the ingredients are well combined.
- In a separate bowl, whisk together balsamic vinegar and olive oil to create the dressing. Drizzle the dressing over the farro salad and toss to coat. Season the salad with additional salt and pepper according to your taste.
- Garnish the salad with fresh cilantro leaves and a squeeze of lemon juice. Serve the Warm Roasted Vegetable Farro Salad as a delicious and nutritious meal.

Nutritional Info: Calories: 298kcal, Carbohydrates: 53g, Protein: 8g, Fat: 8g, Saturated Fat: 1g, Sodium: 896mg, Potassium: 638mg, Fiber: 10g, Sugar: 9g, Vitamin A: 712IU, Vitamin C: 20mg, Calcium: 162mg, Iron: 2mg

4. Roasted Broccoli with Lemon Garlic & Toasted Pine Nuts

(Ready in: 22mins| Serves: 4)

Ingredients:

- 1 lb broccoli florets
- Salt & freshly ground black pepper
- 2 tablespoons olive oil
- 2 tablespoons unsalted butter
- 1/2 teaspoon lemon zest, grated
- 1 teaspoon garlic, minced
- 1-2 tablespoons fresh lemon juice
- 2 tablespoons pine nuts, toasted

Instructions:

- Preheat the oven to 500°F (260°C).
- Toss the broccoli with olive oil in a wide bowl and season with salt and pepper to taste.

- Arrange the broccoli florets in a single layer on a baking sheet and roast, turning once, for 12 minutes or until just tender.
- Meanwhile, melt the butter in a small saucepan over medium heat. Add the grated lemon zest and minced garlic and cook for about 1 minute, stirring.
- Let the lemon butter cool slightly and then stir in the fresh lemon juice.
- Place the roasted broccoli in a serving bowl, pour the lemon butter over it, and toss to coat the broccoli evenly.
- Sprinkle the toasted pine nuts over the top.
- Serve the roasted broccoli with lemon, garlic, and toasted pine nuts as a delightful and nutritious side dish.

Nutritional Info: Calories: 227 kcal, Protein: 6g, Carbohydrates: 12g, Fat: 19g, Sodium: 101mg

5. Creamy Black Bean Soup

(Ready in: 25 mins | Serves: 4)

Ingredients:

- 3 tablespoons olive oil
- 1 tablespoon ground cumin
- 1 medium onion, chopped
- 2-3 cloves garlic, minced
- 2 (14 1/2 ounce) cans black beans, drained and rinsed
- Salt and pepper, to taste
- 2 cups vegetable broth
- 1 small red onion, finely chopped
- 1/4 cup cilantro, coarsely chopped

Instructions:

- In a large pot, heat olive oil over medium heat. Add chopped onion and sauté until translucent. Stir in ground cumin and cook for 30 seconds, then add minced garlic and cook for an additional 30 to 60 seconds until fragrant.
- Add one can of black beans and the vegetable broth to the pot. Bring the mixture to a boil, then reduce heat and simmer for about 10 minutes, stirring occasionally.
- Using a hand blender or a regular blender, puree the soup until smooth and creamy. Return the pureed soup to the pot.
- Add the second can of black beans to the pot and stir to combine. Simmer the soup for another 5-10 minutes to allow the flavors to meld. Season with salt and pepper to taste.

- Serve the creamy black bean soup in bowls, garnishing each serving with chopped red onion and cilantro.

Nutritional Info: Calories: 236 kcal, Protein: 8g, Carbohydrates: 29g, Fat: 11g, Fiber: 9g

---

6. Lentil Veggie Burgers

(Ready in: 1hr 10mins | Yield: 8-10 burgers)

Ingredients:

- 2 1/2 cups water
- 1 cup dry lentils, well rinsed
- 1/2 teaspoon salt
- 1/2 medium onion, diced
- 1 carrot, diced
- 1 tablespoon olive oil
- 1 teaspoon pepper
- 1 tablespoon soy sauce
- 3/4 cup breadcrumbs
- 3/4 cup rolled oats, finely ground

Instructions:

- In a saucepan, bring the water to a boil and add the rinsed lentils and salt. Reduce the heat to a simmer and cook the lentils for about 45 minutes until they are soft and most of the water is absorbed.
- In a separate pan, heat olive oil over medium heat and sauté the diced onion and carrot until tender, about 5 minutes.
- In a large mixing bowl, combine the cooked lentils, sautéed onions and carrots, pepper, soy sauce, breadcrumbs, and finely ground rolled oats. Mix well to form a cohesive mixture.
- While the mixture is still warm, shape it into 8-10 burger patties. You can either shallow fry the lentil burgers on each side for 1-2 minutes or bake them in a preheated oven at 200°C for 15 minutes until they are golden and crispy on the outside.
- Serve the hearty lentil veggie burgers in buns with your favorite toppings and condiments.

Nutritional Info: Calories: 193 kcal, Protein: 8g, Carbohydrates: 31g, Fat: 4g, Fiber: 7g

7. BBQ Chicken Tostadas

(Prep Time: 10 mins | Cook Time: 8 mins | Servings: 4)

Ingredients:

- 3 cups cooked and shredded chicken
- 1 1/2 cups of your favorite barbecue sauce, divided
- 8 tostada shells or 8 corn tortillas brushed lightly with olive oil and baked for 3-5 minutes per side, until crispy
- 3 green onions, very thinly sliced (optional)
- 2 cups shredded cheese (cheddar, Monterey Jack, or a blend)

Instructions:

- Preheat your oven to 350°F. Arrange the tostada shells (or baked tortillas) on two rimmed baking sheets.
- In a small bowl, mix the shredded chicken with 1 cup of barbecue sauce, and toss to coat.
- Divide the chicken evenly between the tostada shells and top with shredded cheese (about 1/4 cup each).
- Bake the tostadas for 6 to 8 minutes, just until the cheese is melted.
- Remove from the oven and drizzle with the remaining 1/2 cup of barbecue sauce.
- Sprinkle with thinly sliced green onions, if desired.

Nutritional Info: 563 kcal | Carbohydrates: 57g | Protein: 42g | Fat: 17g | Saturated Fat: 8g | Cholesterol: 108mg | Sodium: 1370mg | Potassium: 336mg | Fiber: 2g | Sugar: 25g | Vitamin A: 808IU | Vitamin C: 2mg | Calcium: 433mg | Iron: 2mg

8. Buffalo Chicken Sandwich with Blue Cheese Slaw

(Prep Time: 15 mins | Cook Time: 10 mins | Servings: 4)

Ingredients:

Blue Cheese Slaw:

- 1/4 cup mayonnaise
- 1 tablespoon minced garlic
- 1/4 cup crumbled blue cheese
- 2 tablespoons Worcestershire sauce
- 1 (10-ounce) package coleslaw mix
- Kosher salt
- 1 lemon, juiced

- Freshly cracked black pepper

Buffalo Chicken:
- 1/2 cup buffalo hot sauce
- 2 tablespoons smoked paprika, plus more for seasoning
- 4 (6-ounce) boneless, skinless chicken cutlets
- 1 tablespoon kosher salt, plus more for seasoning
- 1 cup self-rising flour
- 1 1/4 cups buttermilk
- 2 tablespoons hot sauce
- 1 egg
- 1 tablespoon cracked black pepper, plus more for seasoning
4 soft club rolls, split and toasted

Instructions:
- In a medium-sized bowl, mix the mayonnaise, crumbled blue cheese, minced garlic, Worcestershire sauce, lemon juice, salt, and freshly cracked black pepper. Add the coleslaw mix and toss well. Set aside.
- Heat enough canola oil in a deep-fryer or heavy-bottomed pot to come halfway up the sides of the pot to 350 degrees F. In a shallow dish, add the buffalo hot sauce and set aside.
- the chicken with smoked paprika, salt, and pepper to taste. In another shallow dish, place the flour, two tablespoons of paprika, one tablespoon of salt, and one tablespoon of pepper. In a separate shallow dish, whisk together the egg, buttermilk, and hot sauce. Dredge each piece of chicken in the flour mixture, then shake off any excess, dip it into the buttermilk mixture, and finally dredge it again in the flour mixture.
- Fry the chicken until cooked through, about 4 to 6 minutes, or until it reaches an internal temperature of 165 degrees F. Dip the cooked chicken into the buffalo hot sauce and place it on the toasted club rolls.
- Top the chicken with a generous amount of blue cheese slaw, and serve.

Nutritional Info: Calories: 712 kcal | Carbohydrates: 57g | Protein: 40g | Fat: 36g | Saturated Fat: 11g | Cholesterol: 135mg | Sodium: 2681mg | Potassium: 482mg | Fiber: 4g | Sugar: 8g | Vitamin A: 1490IU | Vitamin C: 22mg | Calcium: 370mg | Iron: 4mg

9. Oriental Turkey Burger
(Prep Time: 10 min | Cook Time: 20-30 min | Servings: 4)

Ingredients:

Ingredients:
SLAW:

- 2 cups coleslaw mix
- 1 tablespoon seasoned rice vinegar
- 3 tablespoons chopped fresh cilantro
- 1 teaspoon vegetable oil

BURGER:
- 2 tablespoons butter
- 2 jalapeño chile peppers, seeded, finely chopped
- 1/3 cup chopped green onions
- 1 1/4 pounds lean ground turkey
- 1 tablespoon hoisin sauce
- 1 tablespoon soy sauce
- 1/4 cup dry bread crumbs
- 1 tablespoon melted butter
- Hoisin sauce (if desired)
- 5 (10-inch) tortillas

Instructions:
- Heat the gas grill or charcoal grill until the coals are ash white and hot on medium heat. In a bowl, mix all the slaw ingredients; toss well. Cover and let it cool until serving time.
- Melt 2 tablespoons of butter until sizzling in a 10-inch skillet; add the green onions and jalapeño peppers. Cook for about 1-2 minutes or until tender. Set aside to cool. In a bowl, combine the onion mixture, ground turkey, bread crumbs, hoisin sauce, and soy sauce; mix gently. Shape into four patties (3/4 inch thick).
- Place the patties on the grill and brush with melted butter. Grill for about 20-30 minutes, rotating once, or until the internal temperature reaches a minimum of 165°F (74°C) and the center of the meat is no longer pink.
- Wrap the tortillas in aluminum foil and place them away from direct heat on the grill. Rotate the tortillas often while grilling the burgers.
- Top each warm tortilla with a turkey burger. Add slaw and drizzle with hoisin sauce, if desired. Fold the tortilla over the burger to form an Oriental turkey burger.

Nutritional Info: Calories 438, Protein 25g, Carbohydrates 34g, Fat 21g, Saturated Fat 6g, Sodium 700mg, Fiber 4g, Sugar 3g, Vitamin A 70IU, Vitamin C 9mg, Calcium 59mg, Iron 3mg.

10. Shrimp Diablo Spaghetti

(Prep Time: 5 minutes | Cook Time: 25 minutes | Servings: 4)

Ingredients:

- 1/2 teaspoon olive oil
- 1/2 onion, chopped
- 3 cloves garlic, crushed
- 1/2 green bell pepper, chopped
- 1/2 yellow bell pepper, chopped
- 1 can diced tomatoes
- 1/4 cup white wine
- 1/4 teaspoon red pepper flakes
- 1/4 teaspoon dried oregano
- 1/4 teaspoon dried basil
- Salt and ground black pepper to taste
- 6 ounces cooked shrimp
- 4 ounces spaghetti
- 1/4 cup grated Pecorino-Romano cheese
- 1/4 cup chopped fresh parsley, divided

Instructions:

- In a Dutch oven, heat olive oil over medium-high heat. Add chopped yellow bell pepper, green bell pepper, onions, and garlic. Sauté until softened, about 5 to 7 minutes. Season with salt and pepper.
- Stir in the diced tomatoes, white wine, 1/4 cup parsley, oregano, basil, and red pepper flakes. Lower the heat to low, cover the Dutch oven, and cook, stirring occasionally, for about 20 minutes or until the tomatoes break down.
- In a separate large saucepan, bring salted water to a boil. Cook the spaghetti according to package instructions until al dente. Add the cooked shrimp to the sauce and continue cooking for an additional 2 to 4 minutes until the shrimp are fully heated.
- Drain the spaghetti and add it to the sauce with the shrimp. Toss everything together to coat the spaghetti with the sauce. Sprinkle with grated Pecorino-Romano cheese and the remaining parsley before serving.

Nutritional Info: Calories: 303 kcal | Carbohydrates: 38g | Protein: 17g | Fat: 8g | Saturated Fat: 3g | Cholesterol: 59mg | Sodium: 265mg | Potassium: 394mg | Fiber: 3g | Sugar: 3g | Vitamin A: 805IU | Vitamin C: 49mg | Calcium: 111mg | Iron: 2mg

11. Grilled Lemon Herb Salmon

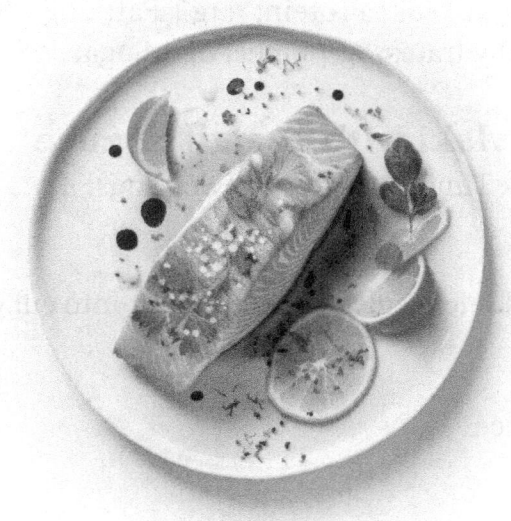

(Prep Time: 10 minutes | Cook Time: 12 minutes | Servings: 4)

Ingredients:

- 4 salmon fillets (about 6 ounces each)
- 2 tablespoons olive oil
- 2 tablespoons fresh lemon juice
- 2 cloves garlic, minced
- 1 teaspoon dried thyme
- 1 teaspoon dried rosemary
- 1 teaspoon dried oregano
- Salt and pepper to taste
- Lemon wedges and fresh parsley for garnish

Instructions:

- Preheat the grill to medium-high heat.
- In a small bowl, whisk together olive oil, lemon juice, minced garlic, dried thyme, dried rosemary, dried oregano, salt, and pepper.
- Place the salmon fillets in a shallow dish and pour the marinade over them. Make sure the fillets are coated evenly. Let them marinate for about 10 minutes.

- Grease the grill grates with some olive oil to prevent sticking. Place the marinated salmon fillets on the grill and cook for about 5-6 minutes on each side, or until the salmon is cooked through and easily flakes with a fork.
- Remove the salmon from the grill and garnish with lemon wedges and fresh parsley before serving.

Nutritional Info: Calories: 340kcal | Protein: 34g | Fat: 20g | Saturated Fat: 3g | Cholesterol: 94mg | Sodium: 89mg | Carbohydrates: 1g | Fiber: 0g | Sugar: 0g

12. Greek Chicken Souvlaki with Tzatziki Sauce

(Prep Time: 20 minutes | Cook Time: 10 minutes | Servings: 4)

Ingredients:

- 1 ½ pounds boneless, skinless chicken breasts, cut into cubes
- ¼ cup olive oil
- 2 tablespoons lemon juice
- 2 cloves garlic, minced
- 1 teaspoon dried oregano
- ½ teaspoon dried thyme
- Salt and pepper to taste
- Wooden skewers, soaked in water
- Tzatziki sauce for serving (store-bought or homemade)

Instructions:

- In a bowl, combine olive oil, lemon juice, minced garlic, dried oregano, dried thyme, salt, and pepper. Add the chicken cubes and toss to coat them evenly. Cover the bowl and let the chicken marinate in the fridge for at least 1 hour.
- Preheat the grill to medium-high heat.
- Thread the marinated chicken cubes onto the soaked wooden skewers.
- Grill the chicken skewers for about 4-5 minutes on each side, or until the chicken is cooked through and has nice grill marks.
- Serve the Greek Chicken Souvlaki with tzatziki sauce on the side for dipping.

Nutritional Info: Calories: 271kcal | Protein: 34g | Fat: 13g | Saturated Fat: 2g | Cholesterol: 96mg | Sodium: 90mg | Carbohydrates: 1g | Fiber: 0g | Sugar: 0g

13. Zucchini Noodles with Pesto and Cherry Tomatoes

(Prep Time: 15 minutes | Cook Time: 5 minutes| Servings: 4)

Ingredients:

- 4 medium zucchinis, spiralized into noodles
- 1 cup cherry tomatoes, halved
- ¼ cup pine nuts, toasted
- Grated Parmesan cheese for serving (optional)

For Pesto:

- 2 cups fresh basil leaves
- ½ cup grated Parmesan cheese
- ½ cup extra-virgin olive oil
- ¼ cup pine nuts
- 2 cloves garlic
- Salt and pepper to taste

Instructions:

- In a food processor, combine all the pesto ingredients and blend until smooth. Season with salt and pepper to taste.
- In a large pan, sauté the zucchini noodles over medium heat for about 2-3 minutes, until they are just tender. Avoid overcooking to keep the noodles al dente. Add the halved cherry tomatoes to the pan and cook for another minute to warm them up. Toss the zucchini noodles and cherry tomatoes with the prepared pesto sauce.
- Serve the zucchini noodles with toasted pine nuts and grated Parmesan cheese on top, if desired.

Nutritional Info: Calories: 306kcal | Protein: 7g | Fat: 29g | Saturated Fat: 5g | Cholesterol: 7mg | Sodium: 75mg | Carbohydrates: 8g | Fiber: 2g | Sugar: 5g

14. Spicy Thai Shrimp Salad with Peanut Dressing

(Prep Time: 15 minutes | Cook Time: 5 minutes | Servings: 4)

Ingredients:

- 1 pound large shrimp, peeled and deveined
- 2 cups mixed salad greens
- 1 cup shredded red cabbage
- 1 cup shredded carrots

- 1 red bell pepper, thinly sliced
- ¼ cup chopped cilantro
- ¼ cup chopped peanuts
- Lime wedges for serving

For Peanut Dressing:
- ¼ cup peanut butter
- 2 tablespoons soy sauce
- 2 tablespoons lime juice
- 1 tablespoon honey
- 1 tablespoon sesame oil
- 1 teaspoon grated ginger
- 1 clove garlic, minced
- 1 teaspoon sriracha sauce (adjust to taste)
- 2 tablespoons water (adjust for desired consistency)

Instructions:
- In a small bowl, whisk together all the ingredients for the peanut dressing until smooth. Adjust the consistency with water as needed. Season the shrimp with salt and pepper. In a pan over medium-high heat, cook the shrimp for about 2-3 minutes per side until they are pink and cooked through.
- In a large bowl, combine the mixed salad greens, shredded red cabbage, shredded carrots, and sliced red bell pepper.
- Add the cooked shrimp to the salad and toss with the prepared peanut dressing.
- Garnish the salad with chopped cilantro, chopped peanuts, and lime wedges.

Nutritional Info: Calories: 342kcal | Protein: 28g | Fat: 20g | Saturated Fat: 3g | Cholesterol: 214mg | Sodium: 796mg | Carbohydrates: 16g | Fiber: 4g | Sugar: 8g

15. Moroccan Chickpea Stew with Quinoa
(Prep Time: 10 minutes | Cook Time: 25 minutes | Servings: 4)

Ingredients:
- 1 tablespoon olive oil
- 1 large onion, chopped
- 2 cloves garlic, minced
- 1 teaspoon ground cumin

- 1 teaspoon ground coriander
- ½ teaspoon ground cinnamon
- ½ teaspoon ground turmeric
- 1 cup canned diced tomatoes
- 2 cups cooked chickpeas
- 3 cups vegetable broth
- ½ cup dried apricots, chopped
- ½ cup chopped dried figs
- 2 cups cooked quinoa
- Fresh cilantro for garnish

Instructions:
- In a large pot, heat the olive oil over medium heat. Add the chopped onion and cook until it becomes soft and translucent. Stir in the minced garlic, ground cumin, ground coriander, ground cinnamon, and ground turmeric. Cook for another minute until fragrant.
- Add the canned diced tomatoes, cooked chickpeas, and vegetable broth to the pot. Bring to a simmer and let it cook for about 10 minutes.
- Stir in the chopped dried apricots and chopped dried figs. Let the stew simmer for an additional 10-15 minutes until the flavors meld together.
- Serve the Moroccan chickpea stew over cooked quinoa and garnish with fresh cilantro.

Nutritional Info: Calories: 390kcal | Protein: 12g | Fat: 7g | Saturated Fat: 1g | Cholesterol: 0mg | Sodium: 637mg | Carbohydrates: 75g | Fiber: 14g | Sugar: 29g

16. Teriyaki Tofu and Vegetable Skewers
(Prep Time: 20 minutes | Cook Time: 15 minutes | Servings: 4)

Ingredients:
- 1 block firm tofu, cut into cubes
- 1 red bell pepper, cut into chunks
- 1 yellow bell pepper, cut into chunks
- 1 zucchini, sliced into rounds
- 1 cup cherry tomatoes
- ¼ cup teriyaki sauce (store-bought or homemade)
- Wooden skewers, soaked in water

Instructions:
- Preheat the grill to medium-high heat.
- Thread the tofu cubes, red bell pepper chunks, yellow bell pepper chunks, zucchini rounds, and cherry tomatoes onto the soaked wooden skewers, alternating between the ingredients.
- Brush the teriyaki sauce over the skewers, making sure to coat all the vegetables and tofu evenly. Grill the skewers for about 6-8 minutes, turning them occasionally, until the tofu and vegetables are charred and cooked through.
- Serve the teriyaki tofu and vegetable skewers with a side of brown rice or quinoa, if desired.

Nutritional Info: Nutritional Information per serving (without rice or quinoa): Calories: 190kcal | Protein: 12g | Fat: 9g | Saturated Fat: 1g | Cholesterol: 0mg | Sodium: 620mg | Carbohydrates: 18g | Fiber: 4g | Sugar: 11g

17. Mediterranean Zoodle Bowl with Olives and Feta

(Prep Time: 15 minutes | Cook Time: 5 minutes | Servings: 4)

Ingredients:
- 4 medium zucchinis, spiralized into noodles
- 1 cup cherry tomatoes, halved
- ½ cup pitted Kalamata olives, sliced
- ½ cup crumbled feta cheese
- ¼ cup chopped fresh parsley
- 2 tablespoons extra-virgin olive oil
- 2 tablespoons red wine vinegar
- 1 teaspoon dried oregano
- Salt and pepper to taste

Instructions:
- In a large bowl, combine the spiralized zucchini noodles, halved cherry tomatoes, sliced Kalamata olives, crumbled feta cheese, and chopped fresh parsley.
- In a small bowl, whisk together the extra-virgin olive oil, red wine vinegar, dried oregano, salt, and pepper to make the dressing.
- Pour the dressing over the zoodle bowl and toss everything together until well combined.
- Serve the Mediterranean zoodle bowl as a refreshing and light lunch option.

Nutritional Info: Calories: 180 kcal, Protein: 6g, Fat: 13g, Carbohydrates: 11g

Fiber: 3g, Sugar: 7g, Sodium: 450mg

18. Lemon Garlic Shrimp and Asparagus Stir-Fry

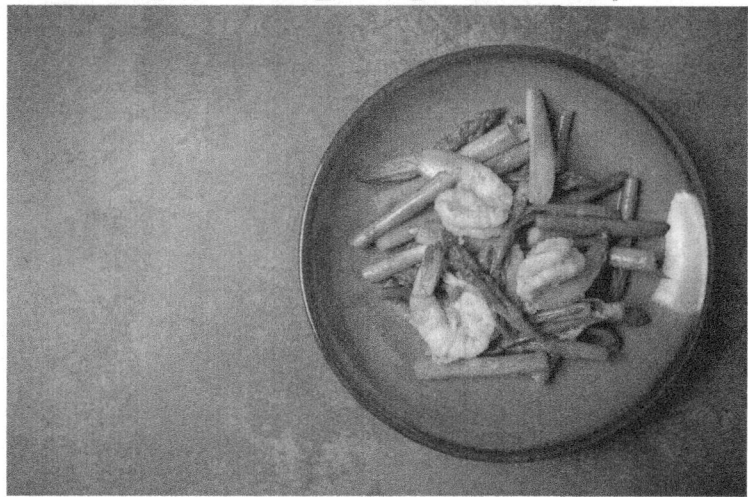

(Prep Time: 10 minutes | Cook Time: 10 minutes | Servings: 4)

Ingredients:

- 1 pound large shrimp, peeled and deveined
- 1 bunch asparagus, trimmed and cut into bite-sized pieces
- 2 tablespoons olive oil
- 4 cloves garlic, minced
- Juice of 1 lemon
- Zest of 1 lemon
- Salt and pepper to taste
- Fresh parsley for garnish

Instructions:

- In a large skillet or wok, heat the olive oil over medium-high heat.
- Add the minced garlic and sauté for about 1 minute until fragrant.
- Add the asparagus to the skillet and stir-fry for 2-3 minutes until tender-crisp.
- Push the asparagus to the side of the skillet and add the shrimp to the center. Cook the shrimp for about 2 minutes per side until they turn pink and opaque.
- Drizzle the lemon juice and lemon zest over the shrimp and asparagus. Season with salt and pepper to taste.
- Garnish with fresh parsley before serving.

Nutritional Info: Calories: 220 kcal, Protein: 25g, Fat: 10g, Carbohydrates: 8g, Fiber: 3g, Sugar: 2g, Sodium: 300mg

19. Asian Sesame Chicken Salad

(Prep Time: 15 minutes | Cook Time: 10 minutes | Servings: 4)

Ingredients:

- 1 pound boneless, skinless chicken breasts
- 8 cups mixed salad greens
- 1 cup shredded carrots
- 1 cucumber, thinly sliced
- 1/4 cup sliced almonds
- 2 tablespoons sesame seeds
- 1/4 cup sesame oil
- 2 tablespoons soy sauce
- 2 tablespoons rice vinegar
- 1 tablespoon honey
- 1 clove garlic, minced
- 1 teaspoon grated ginger
- Fresh cilantro for garnish

Instructions:

- Season the chicken breasts with salt and pepper. Grill or cook the chicken in a skillet over medium heat until it is cooked through and no longer pink in the center, about 4-5 minutes per side. Let it rest for a few minutes before slicing.
- In a large salad bowl, combine the mixed greens, shredded carrots, and cucumber slices.
- Top the salad with the sliced chicken, sliced almonds, and sesame seeds.
- In a small bowl, whisk together the sesame oil, soy sauce, rice vinegar, honey, minced garlic, and grated ginger to make the dressing.
- Drizzle the dressing over the salad and toss to coat evenly. Garnish the Asian sesame chicken salad with fresh cilantro before serving.

Nutritional Info: Calories: 320 kcal, Protein: 25g, Fat: 18g, Carbohydrates: 14g, Fiber: 4g, Sugar: 8g, Sodium: 420mg

20. Roasted Vegetable Quinoa Bowl with Tahini Dressing

(Prep Time: 15 minutes | Cook Time: 25 minutes | Servings: 4)

Ingredients:

- 1 cup quinoa, rinsed
- 2 cups mixed vegetables (e.g., bell peppers, zucchini, eggplant, cherry tomatoes)
- 2 tablespoons olive oil
- 1 teaspoon dried oregano
- Salt and pepper to taste
- 1/4 cup chopped fresh parsley
- 1/4 cup crumbled feta cheese
- 1/4 cup tahini
- 2 tablespoons lemon juice
- 1 clove garlic, minced
- Water (to adjust the consistency)

Instructions:

- Preheat the oven to 400°F (200°C).
- In a saucepan, cook the quinoa according to package instructions. Set aside.
- In a large baking dish, toss the mixed vegetables with olive oil, dried oregano, salt, and pepper.
- Roast the vegetables in the oven for about 20 minutes or until they are tender and slightly charred.
- In a small bowl, whisk together the tahini, lemon juice, minced garlic, and water until it forms a smooth and creamy dressing. Add water as needed to adjust the consistency.
- In serving bowls, assemble the roasted vegetables on a bed of cooked quinoa.
- Drizzle the tahini dressing over the quinoa bowl.
- Garnish with chopped fresh parsley and crumbled feta cheese.

Nutritional Info: Calories: 380 kcal, Protein: 12g, Fat: 26g, Carbohydrates: 30g, Fiber: 6g, Sugar: 4g, Sodium: 60mg

Chapter 5: Dinner Recipes For Intermittent Fasting

1. Cajun Potato, Prawn/Shrimp, and Avocado Salad

(Ready in: 30mins | Serves: 2)

Ingredients:

- 1 tablespoon olive oil
- 300g new potatoes (small baby or chats), halved (10 oz)
- 250g king prawns (shrimp), cooked and peeled (8 oz)
- 2 spring onions, finely sliced
- 1 garlic clove, minced
- 2 teaspoons Cajun seasoning
- 1 cup alfalfa sprouts
- 1 avocado, peeled, stoned, and diced
- Salt (for boiling potatoes)

Instructions:

1. Cook the halved new potatoes in a large saucepan of lightly salted boiling water for 10 to 15 minutes or until tender. Drain the potatoes well.
2. In a wok or large nonstick frying pan/skillet, heat the olive oil over medium-high heat. Add the cooked and peeled prawns, minced garlic, sliced spring onions, and Cajun seasoning. Stir-fry for 2 to 3 minutes until the prawns are heated through and coated with the seasoning.
3. Add the drained new potatoes to the wok and stir them in with the prawns, ensuring they are well combined. Cook for an additional minute to let the flavors meld.
4. Transfer the Cajun potato and prawn mixture to serving dishes.
5. Top the salad with diced avocado and a generous amount of alfalfa sprouts for added freshness and texture.
6. Serve the Cajun Potato, Prawn, and Avocado Salad immediately and enjoy this flavorful and nutritious dish.

Nutritional Info: Calories: 495 kcal, Carbohydrates: 43g, Protein: 27g, Fat: 26g, Saturated Fat: 4g, Fiber: 13g, Sugar: 3g, Sodium: 522mg

2. Cauliflower Pizza Crust

(Ready in: 1hr 10mins | Serves: 4)

Ingredients:

- One egg, beaten
- Four cups raw cauliflower, riced, or one medium cauliflower head
- One cup chevre cheese or 1 cup other soft cheese
- One pinch salt
- One teaspoon dried oregano

Instructions:

1. Preheat your oven to 400°F (200°C). Pulse batches of raw cauliflower florets in a food processor until they resemble a rice-like texture. Fill a large pot with about an inch of water and bring it to a boil. Place the cauliflower rice in a fine-mesh strainer and then submerge it in the boiling water. Cook for about 5 minutes. Drain the cauliflower rice and transfer it to a clean, thin dishtowel. Wrap the dishtowel around the rice, squeezing out excess moisture. This step is crucial to achieving a dry crust for your pizza.

2. In a large bowl, mix the strained cauliflower rice, beaten egg, chevre cheese, salt, and dried oregano. Use your hands to thoroughly combine the ingredients until it forms a dough-like consistency.

3. Line a baking sheet with parchment paper. Place the cauliflower mixture on the parchment paper and press it out into a circle, creating a pizza crust. Keep the crust about 3/8" thick, and make the edges slightly higher for a crust effect if desired.

4. Bake the crust in the preheated oven for 35-40 minutes or until it becomes golden brown and firm. Once the crust is ready, add your favorite pizza sauce, cheese, and any other toppings you desire. Return the pizza to the oven, now set at 400°F (200°C), and bake for an additional 5-10 minutes, or until the cheese is melted and bubbly.

Nutritional Info: Calories: 164 kcal, Protein: 9g, Carbohydrates: 9g, Fat: 10g.

3. Sweet Potato Curry With Spinach And Chickpeas

(Preparation Time: 30 minutes | Serving 6)

Ingredients:

- 1-2 teaspoons canola oil
- 1 tablespoon cumin
- 2 tablespoons curry powder
- 1 teaspoon cinnamon
- 1/2 large sweet onion, chopped, or 2 scallions, thinly sliced

- 10 ounces fresh spinach, washed, stemmed, and coarsely chopped
- 1 (14 1/2-ounce) can chickpeas, rinsed and drained
- 2 large sweet potatoes, peeled and diced (about 2 lbs)
- 1/2 cup water
- 1/4 cup chopped fresh cilantro for garnish
- 1 (14 1/2-ounce) can diced tomatoes, or fresh if available
- Basmati rice or brown rice, for serving

Instructions:

- Heat 1-2 teaspoons of canola or vegetable oil in a large saucepan over medium heat. Add the onions and sauté for 2-3 minutes, or until tender.
- Stir in the curry powder, cumin, and cinnamon, and cook for another 2-3 minutes to evenly coat the onions with the spices.
- Add the diced tomatoes with their juices and stir in the chickpeas. Pour in 1/2 cup of water and bring to a high simmer for 1-2 minutes.
- Add the fresh spinach, a few handfuls at a time, stirring to wilt it. Cover and cook for about 3 minutes until all the spinach is added and wilted.
- Stir in the cooked sweet potatoes, coating them with the flavorful mixture. Simmer for an additional 3-5 minutes to blend the flavors.
- Transfer to a serving dish, garnish with fresh cilantro, and serve over basmati or brown rice.

Nutritional Info: Calories: 241 kcal, Protein: 6g, Carbohydrates: 42g, Fat: 6g.

4. Vegan Fried 'Fish' Tacos

(Ready in: 50 mins | Yield: 8 small tacos)

Ingredients:

- 14 ounces silken tofu
- 1/2 cup plain flour
- 2 cups panko breadcrumbs
- 1/2 teaspoon salt
- 1/2 teaspoon cayenne pepper
- 1 teaspoon smoked paprika
- 1 teaspoon ground cumin
- 1/2 cup non-dairy milk
- 1/4 head cabbage, finely shredded

- Vegetable oil, for frying
- 1 ripe avocado
- Vegan mayonnaise, to serve
- 8 small tortillas

Pickled Onion:

- 1 red onion, peeled, finely sliced
- 1 tablespoon sugar
- 1/4 cup apple cider vinegar
- 1 teaspoon salt

Instructions:

- Pat the tofu with a few pieces of kitchen roll to extract excess moisture. Cut the tofu into rough 1-inch pieces.
- Place the panko breadcrumbs in a shallow, large cup. In another large, shallow cup, combine the flour, salt, smoked paprika, cayenne, and cumin.
- Pour the non-dairy milk into a third shallow bowl. Coat each piece of tofu first with flour, then dip into the non-dairy milk, and finally, coat with the breadcrumbs.
- Fill a deep frying pan with vegetable oil about 1/2-inch deep. Heat the oil over medium heat until it starts to bubble and brown a breadcrumb when dropped in.
- Fry the breaded tofu in batches until golden underneath, then flip and cook until all sides are golden. Remove to a baking sheet lined with a drainable kitchen roll.
- For the pickled onion: Heat the apple cider vinegar, salt, and sugar in a small pot until steaming. Place the finely sliced red onion in a bowl or pot and pour the hot vinegar over it. Let it sit for at least 30 minutes to soften and turn pink.
- Serve the spicy fried tofu, pickled onion, a smear of vegan mayo, some avocado, and shredded cabbage in warmed tortillas.

Nutritional Info: Calories: 264 kcal, Protein: 7g, Carbohydrates: 26g, Fat: 16g

5. Baked Parmesan Tilapia Delight

(Ready in: 35mins | Serves: 4)

Ingredients:

- 2 lbs tilapia fillets (orange roughy, cod, or red snapper can be substituted)
- 1/2 cup grated parmesan cheese
- 2 tablespoons freshly squeezed lemon juice
- 3 tablespoons mayonnaise

- 3 tablespoons finely chopped green onions
- 4 tablespoons butter, at room temperature
- 1/4 teaspoon dried basil
- Black pepper, to taste
- 1/4 teaspoon seasoning salt (such as Old Bay seasoning)
- A dash of hot pepper sauce

Instructions:

- Preheat the oven to 350°F (175°C). Grease a 13-by-9-inch baking dish or jelly roll pan with butter.
- Lay the tilapia fillets in a single layer in the prepared baking dish, making sure not to stack them.
- Brush the fillets with freshly squeezed lemon juice, coating the top evenly.
- In a mixing bowl, combine the grated parmesan cheese, butter, mayonnaise, finely chopped green onions, dried basil, black pepper, seasoning salt, and a dash of hot pepper sauce. Mix well using a fork until a creamy and well-blended mixture is formed.
- Bake the fish in the preheated oven for 10 to 20 minutes, or until the fish just begins to flake. The baking time will vary depending on the thickness of the fish fillets, so keep an eye on them to prevent overcooking.
- Remove the baking dish from the oven and spread the prepared cheese mixture over the top of the tilapia fillets.
- Return the dish to the oven and bake for an additional 5 minutes, or until the cheese mixture turns golden brown and slightly bubbly.
- Serve the Baked Parmesan Tilapia Delight with your choice of side dishes, such as steamed vegetables or a fresh garden salad.

Nutritional Info: Calories: 330 kcal, Protein: 34g, Carbohydrates: 4g, Fat: 19g, Saturated Fat: 9g, Cholesterol: 120mg, Sodium: 550mg, Fiber: 0.5g, Sugar: 1g

6. Shredded Brussels Sprouts with Bacon and Onions

(Ready in: 30mins | Serves: 6)

Ingredients:

- small yellow onion, thinly sliced
- 2 slices of bacon
- 3/4 cup water
- 1 teaspoon Dijon mustard
- 1/4 teaspoon salt (or to taste)

- 1 tablespoon cider vinegar
- 1 lb Brussels sprouts, trimmed, halved, and very thinly sliced

Instructions:

- In a pan, cook the bacon over medium heat until crisp (5 to 7 minutes). Drain the bacon on paper towels, then crumble it.
- In the same pan with the bacon drippings, add the thinly sliced onion and salt. Cook over medium heat until the onions are tender and browned, stirring frequently (about 3 minutes).
- Add water and Dijon mustard to the pan, scraping any browned bits from the bottom. Add the thinly sliced Brussels sprouts and cook, stirring regularly, until they are tender (4 to 6 minutes).
- Stir in the cider vinegar and add the crumbled bacon on top.
- Serve the shredded Brussels sprouts with bacon and onions as a delicious and flavorful side dish.

Nutritional Info: Calories: 93 kcal, Protein: 4g, Carbohydrates: 9g, Fat: 5g, Sodium: 287mg

7. Sauerkraut Salad

(Preparation Time: 15 minutes | Servings: 6)

Ingredients:

- 1 cup celery, finely chopped
- 1 (1 lb) can sauerkraut, drained but not rinsed
- 1/2 cup green pepper, finely chopped
- 2 tablespoons onions, finely choppe
- 1/3 cup salad oil
- 3/4 cup sugar
- 1/3 cup cider vinegar (or white vinegar)
- 1/2 teaspoon salt
- 1/2 teaspoon pepper

Instructions:

- In a large bowl, mix together the sauerkraut, chopped celery, green pepper, and onions.
- In a saucepan over low heat, heat the sugar, salad oil, vinegar, salt, and pepper until the sugar dissolves.
- Pour the dressing over the sauerkraut mixture and stir to combine.
- Cover the bowl and refrigerate the sauerkraut salad overnight to allow the flavors to meld.

Nutritional Info: Calories: 180 kcal, Protein: 1g, Carbohydrates: 29g, Fat: 7g

8. Vegetable Turkey Meatloaf with Balsamic Glaze

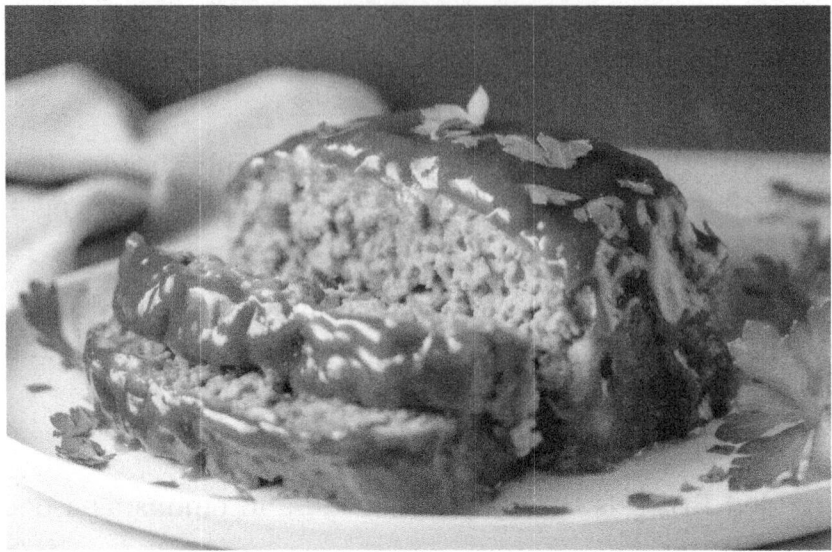

(Prep Time: 20 mins | Cook Time: 1 hr 15 mins | Servings: 6)

Ingredients:

- 2 tablespoons extra-virgin olive oil
- 1 small zucchini, finely diced
- 1 large egg, lightly beaten
- 1 red bell pepper, finely diced
- 1 yellow bell pepper, finely diced
- 5 cloves garlic, smashed to a paste with coarse salt
- Kosher salt and freshly ground pepper
- 1/4 cup chopped fresh parsley
- 1/2 cup grated Parmesan cheese or freshly grated Romano
- 1 1/2 pounds ground turkey (90% lean)
- 1 cup panko (coarse Japanese breadcrumbs)
- 1 tablespoon finely chopped fresh thyme
- 1/4 cup plus two tablespoons balsamic vinegar
- 3/4 cup ketchup

Instructions:

- Preheat the oven to 425°F. In a large sauté pan, heat 1/2 tablespoon of olive oil over medium-high heat. Add the onions and reduce the heat to medium. Cook, stirring occasionally, until translucent and softened, about 3-5 minutes.

- Add the chopped zucchini, garlic paste, bell peppers, and 1/4 teaspoon of red pepper flakes to the pan. Season with salt and pepper and cook for about 5 minutes until the vegetables are almost tender. Set aside to cool.
- In a large bowl, whisk together the egg and fresh parsley. Add the ground turkey, panko, grated cheese, 1/2 cup of ketchup, two tablespoons of the cooled vegetable mixture, and 1/4 cup of balsamic vinegar. Mix until just combined.
- Gently press the turkey mixture into a 9-by-5-inch loaf pan. In a small bowl, whisk together the remaining 1/4 cup balsamic vinegar, 1/4 cup ketchup, and 1/4 teaspoon red pepper flakes. Brush the glaze over the entire loaf.
- Bake the meatloaf for 1 to 1 1/4 hours or until it reaches an internal temperature of 165°F. Let it rest for 10 minutes before slicing and serving.

Nutritional Info: Calories: 359 kcal | Carbohydrates: 24g | Protein: 25g | Fat: 18g | Saturated Fat: 4g | Cholesterol: 106mg | Sodium: 738mg | Potassium: 582mg | Fiber: 2g | Sugar: 10g | Vitamin A: 1028IU | Vitamin C: 61mg | Calcium: 149mg | Iron: 3mg

9. Italian Chicken

(Cook Time: 30 min | Prep Time: 10 min | Servings: 4)

Ingredients:

- 4 boneless skinless chicken breasts
- 1/2 cup breadcrumbs
- 1/2 cup grated parmesan cheese
- 1/2 teaspoon minced garlic
- Salt and pepper to taste
- 4 tablespoons melted butter
- 1 teaspoon Italian seasoning
- 1 pound small potatoes, halved or quartered
- Cooking spray
- 2 tablespoons chopped parsley
- Lemon wedges (optional, for garnish)

Instructions:

- Preheat the oven to 400°F (200°C) and lightly grease a baking sheet with cooking spray. In a small bowl, mix together the grated parmesan cheese, breadcrumbs, minced garlic, Italian seasoning, salt, and pepper.
- Dip the top of each chicken breast into the melted butter and then press it into the breadcrumb mixture to coat it.

- Place the coated chicken breasts on the prepared baking sheet and scatter the potatoes around them.
- Drizzle the remaining butter over the potatoes and season them with salt and pepper to taste.
- Bake for 25-30 minutes or until the chicken is fully cooked and the potatoes are tender.
- Cooking time may vary depending on the thickness of the chicken.
- Sprinkle with chopped parsley and garnish with lemon wedges, if desired.

Nutritional Info: Calories 375, Protein 36g, Carbohydrates 17g, Fat 18g, Saturated Fat 10g, Sodium 440mg, Fiber 2g, Sugar 1g, Vitamin A 135IU, Vitamin C 14mg, Calcium 204mg, Iron 3mg.

10. Rustic Shepherd's Pie

(Cook time: 50 minutes | Prep time: 15 minutes | Servings: 6)

Ingredients:

- 8 tablespoons (1 stick) butter
- 1 1/2 to 2 pounds potatoes (about three large potatoes), peeled and quartered
- 1 medium onion, chopped (about 1 1/2 cups)
- 1 1/2 lbs ground beef
- 1-2 cups mixed vegetables (diced carrots, corn, peas)
- 1/2 cup beef broth
- Salt, pepper, and other seasonings of choice
- 1 teaspoon Worcestershire sauce

Instructions:

- Boil the potatoes: Place the peeled and quartered potatoes in a medium-sized pot. Cover with cold water, adding a teaspoon of salt. Bring to a boil, then reduce to a simmer and cook until tender (about 20 minutes).
- Sauté vegetables: In a large saucepan, melt four tablespoons of butter over medium heat. Add chopped onions and cook until tender, about 6 to 10 minutes. If using carrots, add them with the onions as they take the same time to cook. For quicker-cooking vegetables like peas or corn, add them later during the cooking process to avoid overcooking.
- Add the ground beef and Worcestershire sauce: Add the ground beef to the pan with onions and vegetables. Cook until no longer pink, and season with salt and pepper. Pour in the beef broth and Worcestershire sauce. Simmer until the liquid reduces, about 10 minutes, adding more beef broth if needed to prevent drying out.

- Mash the cooked potatoes: Once the potatoes are cooked, drain them and transfer to a bowl. Add the remaining four tablespoons of butter and mash with a fork or potato masher. Season with salt and pepper to taste.
- Arrange the meat mixture and mashed potatoes: Preheat the oven to 400°F. Spread the beef, onions, and vegetable mixture in an even layer in a casserole dish. Top with the mashed potatoes, creating peaks with a fork for a golden-brown finish.
- Bake in the oven: Place the casserole dish in the preheated oven and bake for about 30 minutes until the top is browned and bubbling.

Nutritional Info: Calories: 486 kcal | Carbohydrates: 32g | Protein: 25g | Fat: 29g | Saturated Fat: 15g | Cholesterol: 104mg | Sodium: 474mg | Potassium: 1152mg | Fiber: 5g | Sugar: 2g | Vitamin A: 4469IU | Vitamin C: 31mg | Calcium: 70mg | Iron: 7mg

11. Cauliflower Rice Stir-Fry with Tofu and Vegetables

(Prep Time: 15 minutes | Cook Time: 15 minutes | Servings: 4)

Ingredients:

- 1 medium head cauliflower
- 1 block of firm tofu, drained and cubed
- 2 cups mixed vegetables (bell peppers, broccoli, carrots, snap peas, etc.)
- 3 tablespoons soy sauce
- 2 tablespoons sesame oil
- 1 tablespoon rice vinegar
- 1 tablespoon minced garlic
- 1 tablespoon minced ginger
- 2 green onions, chopped
- Sesame seeds and chopped cilantro for garnish

Instructions:

- Grate the cauliflower or pulse in a food processor until it resembles rice. Set aside.
- In a large skillet or wok, heat 1 tablespoon of sesame oil over medium-high heat. Add the cubed tofu and cook until lightly browned. Remove tofu from the skillet and set aside.
- In the same skillet, add another tablespoon of sesame oil and stir-fry the mixed vegetables until tender-crisp.
- Push the vegetables to one side of the skillet and add the remaining tablespoon of sesame oil. Add minced garlic and ginger and cook until fragrant. Add the grated cauliflower to the skillet and stir-fry for 2-3 minutes until tender.
- Return the cooked tofu to the skillet and mix everything together.

- In a small bowl, mix soy sauce and rice vinegar. Pour the sauce over the stir-fry and toss to combine.
- Serve the cauliflower rice stir-fry garnished with chopped green onions, sesame seeds, and cilantro.

Nutritional Info: Calories: 230kcal, Carb: 17g, Protein: 14g, Fat: 13g, Sodium: 520mg

12. Quinoa Stuffed Bell Peppers with Black Beans and Avocado

(Prep Time: 20 minutes | Cook Time: 30 minutes | Servings: 4)

Ingredients:

- 4 large bell peppers (any color)
- 1 cup cooked quinoa
- 1 can (15 oz) black beans, drained and rinsed
- 1 cup diced tomatoes
- 1 cup corn kernels (fresh, frozen, or canned)
- 1/2 cup diced red onion
- 1/2 cup chopped cilantro
- 1 tablespoon olive oil
- 1 tablespoon lime juice
- 1 teaspoon ground cumin
- 1/2 teaspoon chili powder
- Salt and pepper to taste
- Diced avocado for serving

Instructions:

- Preheat the oven to 375°F (190°C).
- Cut the tops off the bell peppers and remove the seeds and membranes. Lightly brush the outside of the peppers with olive oil and place them in a baking dish.
- In a large bowl, mix together cooked quinoa, black beans, diced tomatoes, corn, red onion, cilantro, olive oil, lime juice, ground cumin, chili powder, salt, and pepper.
- Stuff each bell pepper with the quinoa and black bean mixture.
- Cover the baking dish with foil and bake for 25-30 minutes or until the peppers are tender.
- Remove from the oven and let them cool slightly before serving. Top each stuffed pepper with diced avocado before serving.

Nutritional Info: Calories: 330kcal, Carbohydrates: 57g, Protein: 13g, Fat: 8g, Sodium: 420mg

13. Lemon Herb Baked Cod with Steamed Green Beans

(Prep Time: 10 minutes | Cook Time: 15 minutes | Servings: 4)

Ingredients:

- 4 cod fillets (about 6 oz each)
- 1 lemon, sliced
- 2 tablespoons olive oil
- 2 cloves garlic, minced
- 1 tablespoon chopped fresh parsley
- 1 tablespoon chopped fresh dill
- Salt and pepper to taste
- 1 lb fresh green beans, trimmed

Instructions:

- Preheat the oven to 400°F (200°C).
- Place the cod fillets on a baking sheet lined with parchment paper.
- Drizzle olive oil over the cod and rub minced garlic on top.
- Sprinkle chopped parsley and dill over the cod and season with salt and pepper.
- Place lemon slices on top of each fillet.
- Bake in the preheated oven for 12-15 minutes or until the fish flakes easily with a fork.
- While the cod is baking, steam the green beans until tender-crisp, about 5-7 minutes.
- Serve the lemon herb baked cod with steamed green beans on the side.

Nutritional Info: Calories: 300kcal, Carb: 10g, Protein: 35g, Fat: 13g, Sodium: 210mg

14. Ratatouille with Herbed Quinoa

(Prep Time: 20 minutes, Cook Time: 30 minutes, Servings: 4)

Ingredients:

- 1 eggplant, diced
- 1 zucchini, diced
- 1 yellow bell pepper, diced
- 1 red bell pepper, diced
- 1 onion, diced
- 2 cloves garlic, minced
- 2 cups diced tomatoes (canned or fresh)

- 1 tablespoon olive oil
- 1 teaspoon dried thyme
- 1 teaspoon dried oregano
- Salt and pepper to taste
- 1 cup cooked quinoa
- Chopped fresh basil for garnish

Instructions:

- In a large skillet, heat olive oil over medium heat.
- Add diced eggplant, zucchini, yellow bell pepper, red bell pepper, onion, and garlic to the skillet. Cook for 8-10 minutes or until the vegetables are tender.
- Stir in diced tomatoes, dried thyme, dried oregano, salt, and pepper. Simmer for another 5 minutes.
- In a separate pot, cook quinoa according to package instructions.
- Serve the ratatouille over herbed quinoa and garnish with chopped fresh basil.

Nutritional Info: Calories: 230kcal, Carbohydrates: 32g, Protein: 6g, Fat: 9g, Sodium: 280mg

15. Baked Eggplant Parmesan with Mixed Greens Salad

(Prep Time: 20 minutes | Cook Time: 40 minutes | Servings: 4)

Ingredients:

- 1 large eggplant, sliced into 1/2-inch rounds
- 2 cups marinara sauce
- 1 cup whole wheat breadcrumbs
- 1/2 cup grated Parmesan cheese
- 2 eggs, beaten
- 1 tablespoon olive oil
- 4 cups mixed greens (spinach, arugula, kale, etc.)
- 1 tablespoon balsamic vinegar
- 1 tablespoon extra-virgin olive oil
- Salt and pepper to taste

Instructions:

- Preheat the oven to 375°F (190°C).
- Dip each eggplant slice into the beaten eggs and then coat with breadcrumbs. Place the coated eggplant slices on a baking sheet lined with parchment paper.

- Bake in the preheated oven for 20-25 minutes or until the eggplant is tender and golden brown.
- In a separate saucepan, heat marinara sauce over medium heat until warmed through.
- To make the salad, toss mixed greens with balsamic vinegar, extra-virgin olive oil, salt, and pepper.
- Serve the baked eggplant parmesan with warm marinara sauce and a side of mixed greens salad.

Nutritional Info: Calories: 320kcal, Carb: 30g, Protein: 15g, Fat: 15g, Sodium: 670mg

16. Teriyaki Salmon with Sesame Broccoli

(Prep Time: 10 minutes | Cook Time: 15 minutes | Servings: 4)

Ingredients:

- 4 salmon fillets (about 6 oz each)
- 1/4 cup low-sodium soy sauce
- 2 tablespoons honey
- 1 tablespoon rice vinegar
- 2 teaspoons grated fresh ginger
- 2 cloves garlic, minced
- 1 tablespoon sesame oil
- 1 lb fresh broccoli florets
- 1 tablespoon sesame seeds

Instructions:

- In a small bowl, whisk together soy sauce, honey, rice vinegar, grated ginger, and minced garlic to make the teriyaki sauce.
- Place salmon fillets in a shallow dish and pour half of the teriyaki sauce over them. Let them marinate for 10 minutes.
- In a large skillet or wok, heat sesame oil over medium-high heat. Add the marinated salmon fillets and cook for 3-4 minutes on each side, or until cooked through.
- Steam the broccoli florets until tender-crisp, about 5-7 minutes.
- Drizzle the remaining teriyaki sauce over the cooked salmon and sprinkle with sesame seeds.
- Serve the teriyaki salmon with sesame broccoli on the side.

Nutritional Info: Calories: 350kcal, Carb: 18g, Protein: 30g, Fat: 18g, Sodium: 490mg

17. Cilantro Lime Shrimp with Avocado Salsa

(Prep Time: 15 minutes | Cook Time: 5 minutes | Servings: 4)

Ingredients:

- 1 lb large shrimp, peeled and deveined
- 2 tablespoons olive oil
- Zest and juice of 1 lime
- 2 tablespoons chopped fresh cilantro
- Salt and pepper to taste
- 1 avocado, diced
- 1 cup cherry tomatoes, halved
- 1/4 cup diced red onion
- 1 jalapeno, seeded and diced
- 1 tablespoon lime juice
- Salt and pepper to taste

Instructions:

- In a bowl, toss the shrimp with olive oil, lime zest, lime juice, chopped cilantro, salt, and pepper.
- Heat a large skillet over medium-high heat and add the marinated shrimp. Cook for 2-3 minutes on each side, or until pink and opaque.
- In a separate bowl, mix diced avocado, cherry tomatoes, diced red onion, jalapeno, lime juice, salt, and pepper to make the avocado salsa.
- Serve the cilantro lime shrimp with avocado salsa on top.

Nutritional Info: Calories: 240kcal, Carbohydrates: 7g, Protein: 23g, Fat: 14g, Sodium: 390mg

18. Spinach and Mushroom Stuffed Portobello Mushrooms

(Prep Time: 20 minutes | Cook Time: 20 minutes | Servings: 4)

Ingredients:

- 4 large portobello mushrooms
- 2 cups fresh spinach
- 1 cup chopped mushrooms
- 1/2 cup diced onion
- 2 cloves garlic, minced
- 1 tablespoon olive oil

- 1/2 cup shredded mozzarella cheese
- 1/4 cup grated Parmesan cheese
- Salt and pepper to taste

Instructions:

- Preheat the oven to 375°F (190°C).
- Remove the stems and gills from the portobello mushrooms and clean them with a damp cloth.
- In a large skillet, heat olive oil over medium heat. Add chopped mushrooms, diced onion, and minced garlic. Cook until tender.
- Add fresh spinach to the skillet and cook until wilted.
- Season with salt and pepper.
- Stuff each portobello mushroom with the spinach and mushroom mixture.
- Top each stuffed mushroom with shredded mozzarella and grated Parmesan cheese.
- Bake in the preheated oven for 15-20 minutes or until the cheese is melted and bubbly.

Nutritional Info: Calories: 180kcal, Carbohydrates: 8g, Protein: 11g, Fat: 13g, Sodium: 320mg

19. Eggplant and Chickpea Coconut Curry with Brown Rice

(Prep Time: 15 minutes, Cook Time: 30 minutes, Servings: 4)

Ingredients:

- 1 large eggplant, diced
- 1 can (15 oz) chickpeas, drained and rinsed
- 1 can (15 oz) diced tomatoes
- 1 can (13.5 oz) coconut milk
- 1 onion, diced
- 2 cloves garlic, minced
- 1 tablespoon curry powder
- 1 teaspoon ground cumin
- 1/2 teaspoon ground turmeric
- 1 tablespoon olive oil
- Salt and pepper to taste
- 2 cups cooked brown rice
- Chopped fresh cilantro for garnish

Instructions:

- In a large skillet, heat olive oil over medium heat. Add diced eggplant, diced onion, and minced garlic to the skillet. Cook until the eggplant is tender.
- Add chickpeas, diced tomatoes, coconut milk, curry powder, ground cumin, ground turmeric, salt, and pepper to the skillet. Simmer for 10 minutes or until the sauce thickens.
- Serve the eggplant and chickpea coconut curry over cooked brown rice and garnish with chopped fresh cilantro.

Nutritional Info: Calories: 390kcal, Carb: 52g, Protein: 11g, Fat: 16g, Sodium: 460mg

20. Grilled Steak with Chimichurri Sauce and Roasted Sweet Potatoes

(Prep Time: 15 minutes, Cook Time: 25 minutes, Servings: 4)

Ingredients:
- 4 boneless sirloin steaks (about 6 oz each)
- 1/4 cup fresh parsley, chopped
- 2 tablespoons fresh cilantro, chopped
- 2 cloves garlic, minced
- 1/4 cup red wine vinegar
- 1/4 cup extra-virgin olive oil
- 1 teaspoon dried oregano
- Salt and pepper to taste
- 2 large sweet potatoes, peeled and diced
- 1 tablespoon olive oil

Instructions:
- Preheat the grill to medium-high heat. In a small bowl, mix together chopped parsley, chopped cilantro, minced garlic, red wine vinegar, extra-virgin olive oil, dried oregano, salt, and pepper to make the chimichurri sauce. Set aside.
- Rub olive oil, salt, and pepper on both sides of the steaks. Grill the steaks for 3-4 minutes on each side, or until desired doneness. While the steaks are grilling, preheat the oven to 425°F (220°C). Toss diced sweet potatoes with olive oil, salt, and pepper. Spread the sweet potatoes in a single layer on a baking sheet lined with parchment paper.
- Roast the sweet potatoes in the preheated oven for 20 minutes or until tender and golden brown. Serve the grilled steak with chimichurri sauce and roasted sweet potatoes on the side.

Nutritional Info: Calories: 390kcal, Carb: 25g, Protein: 30g, Fat: 18g, Sodium: 250mg

Chapter 6: Snack & Dessert Recipes For Intermittent Fasting

1. Roasted Cauliflower "Popcorn"

(Ready in: 1hr 10mins | Serves: 4)

Ingredients:

- 4 tablespoons olive oil
- 1 head cauliflower
- 1 teaspoon salt, to taste

Instructions:

- Preheat the oven to 425°F (220°C).
- Trim the cauliflower head, removing the thick stems and core. Cut the cauliflower into bite-sized florets, roughly the size of ping-pong balls.
- In a large bowl, whisk together the olive oil and salt. Add the cauliflower florets to the bowl and toss them thoroughly to coat them evenly with the seasoned oil.
- Line a baking sheet with parchment paper (optional) and spread the cauliflower pieces on the sheet.
- Roast the cauliflower in the preheated oven for about 1 hour, turning the florets three or four times during cooking. The cauliflower should turn golden brown and slightly caramelized, enhancing its natural sweetness.

Nutritional Info: Calories: 140 kcal, Protein: 2g, Carbohydrates: 10g, Fat: 11g, Fiber: 4g, Sodium: 597mg

2. Spicy Chocolate Keto Fat Bombs

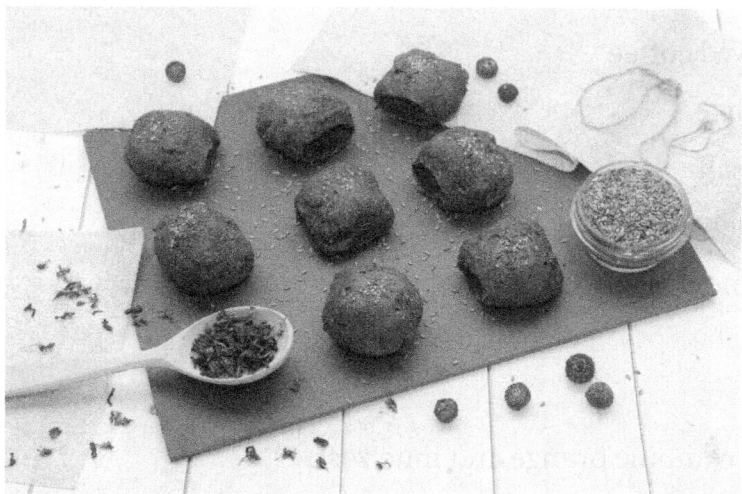

(Preparation Time: 8 minutes | Servings: 24)

Ingredients:

- 2/3 cup coconut oil
- 1/2 cup dark cocoa powder
- 4 (6g) packets stevia (or to taste)
- 2/3 cup smooth peanut butter
- 1 tablespoon ground cinnamon
- 1/2 cup toasted coconut flakes
- 1/4 teaspoon kosher salt
- 1/4 teaspoon cayenne pepper (to taste)

Instructions:

- In a double boiler set over a pot of simmering water, melt the coconut oil, peanut butter, and dark cocoa powder until smooth and well combined.
- Stir in the stevia, ground cinnamon, and kosher salt until fully incorporated.
- Divide the mixture into silicone mini muffin trays.
- Top each fat bomb with toasted coconut flakes and a pinch of cayenne pepper, to add a spicy kick.
- Place the muffin trays in the freezer for about 30 minutes, or until the fat bombs become solid.

Nutritional Info: Calories: 100 kcal, Protein: 2g, Carbohydrates: 3g, Fat: 9g

3. Citrus Dark Chocolate Mousse

(Prep Time: 5 minutes | Cook Time: 15 minutes | Servings: 5)

Ingredients:

- 1 teaspoon brewed coffee
- 85g dark chocolate
- 1 pinch of rock salt
- 1 teaspoon orange zest
- 1/2 teaspoon lime zest
- 3 medium eggs

Instructions:

- In a small dish, combine orange and lime zest.
- In a double boiler, melt the dark chocolate along with the brewed coffee and zest over warm water. Stir to prevent bubbling.

- Remove the melted chocolate from the heat and let it cool.
- In a separate bowl, whisk the egg whites and salt until stiff peaks form. Stir the egg yolks into the cooled chocolate mixture, then gently fold in the whipped egg whites.
- Pour the mousse into small bowls or glasses. Refrigerate for at least 4 hours before serving.

Nutritional Info: Calories: 284kcal | Fat: 20g | Protein: 6g | Sodium: 81mg

4. Peanut Butter Cookies
(Prep Time: 15 minutes | Cook Time: 10 minutes | Servings: 24)

Ingredients:
- 1 cup unsalted butter
- 1 cup crunchy peanut butter
- 1 cup white sugar
- 1 cup packed brown sugar
- 2 large eggs
- 2 1/2 cups all-purpose flour
- 1 teaspoon baking powder
- 1 1/2 teaspoons baking soda
- 1/2 teaspoon salt

Instructions:
- In a mixing bowl, cream together the butter, peanut butter, and both sugars until well combined.
- Add the eggs and continue mixing until smooth. In a separate bowl, whisk together the flour, baking powder, baking soda, and salt.
- Gradually add the dry ingredients to the wet mixture and mix until a dough forms. Refrigerate the dough for 1 hour.
- Preheat the oven to 375°F (190°C) and line baking pans with parchment paper. Roll the dough into 1-inch balls and place them on the prepared baking pans. Use a fork to make a crisscross pattern on each cookie.
- Bake for approximately 10 minutes or until the cookies turn golden brown.
- Allow the cookies to cool on the baking pans for a few minutes before transferring them to a wire rack to cool completely.

Nutritional Info: Calories: 212kcal | Fat: 12g | Protein: 4g | Sodium: 189mg

5. Mango and Passionfruit Roulade

(Prep Time: 20 minutes | Cook Time: 15 minutes | Servings: 4)

Ingredients:

- 3 eggs
- 85g sugar
- 85g plain flour, sifted
- 1 teaspoon baking powder
- 1 teaspoon vanilla extract
- 2 ripe mangoes
- 250g frozen raspberries
- 1 tub of Greek yogurt
- 2 ripe passion fruits

Instructions:

- Preheat the oven to 180°C (350°F) and line a baking pan with parchment paper.
- In a large mixing bowl, whisk the eggs and sugar until thick and light.
- Gently fold in the sifted flour, baking powder, and vanilla extract.
- Pour the batter into the prepared baking pan and spread it evenly.
- Bake for 14-15 minutes until the sponge is lightly browned and springy to the touch.
- While the sponge is still warm, carefully roll it up with the parchment paper inside. Let it cool completely in this rolled-up shape.
- In a separate bowl, mix together the Greek yogurt, one-third of the mangoes (diced), and half of the raspberries.
- Unroll the cooled sponge and spread the yogurt mixture evenly over it. Scatter the remaining diced mangoes and raspberries on top of the yogurt mixture.
- Roll the sponge back up without the parchment paper.
- Cut into slices and serve, garnishing with the pulp of the ripe passion fruits.

Nutritional Info: Calories: 273kcal | Fat: 4g | Protein: 5g | Sodium: 96mg

6. Almond Butter Chocolate Chip Cookies

(Prep Time: 15 minutes | Cook Time: 35 minutes | Servings: 15)

Ingredients:

- ¼ cup chopped peanuts
- 1 egg

- 1 cup almond butter
- ½ cup chocolate chips
- 1 teaspoon baking soda
- ½ cup brown sugar

Instructions:

- Preheat the oven to 350°F (175°C). Line two baking pans with parchment paper.
- In a medium mixing bowl, whisk the egg.
- In another mixing bowl, combine almond butter, brown sugar, and baking soda, and mix until smooth.
- Add the whisked egg to the almond butter mixture and stir until well combined.
- Fold in the chopped peanuts and chocolate chips.
- Using roughly 1 tablespoon of dough for each cookie, roll the dough into compact balls and place them 1 inch apart on the prepared baking pans.
- Gently press down on each ball with the back of a spoon to slightly flatten.
- Bake the cookies for 9 to 10 minutes, or until the tops are cracked and the edges are lightly browned.
- Allow the cookies to cool on the baking pans for 10 minutes before transferring them to a wire rack to cool completely.

Nutritional Info: Fat: 10g; Protein: 4g; Sodium: 108mg

7. Frozen Strawberry-Chocolate Greek Yogurt

(Prep Time: 10 minutes | Freeze Time: 180 minutes | Servings: 32)

Ingredients:

- 1 cup sliced strawberries
- 2 tbsp honey
- ¼ cup chocolate chips
- 3 cups plain Greek yogurt
- 1 teaspoon vanilla extract

Instructions:

- Line a baking sheet with parchment paper.
- In a medium mixing bowl, combine the Greek yogurt, honey, and vanilla extract.
- Spread the yogurt mixture on the lined baking sheet, forming a rectangle.
- Sprinkle the chocolate chips over the yogurt and arrange the sliced strawberries on top.

- Place the baking sheet in the freezer and freeze for at least 3 hours or until the yogurt is extremely firm.
- Once frozen, cut the yogurt into pieces and serve.

Nutritional Info: Fat: 1.3g; Protein: 2g; Sodium: 7.6mg

8. Dark Chocolate Dipped Strawberries

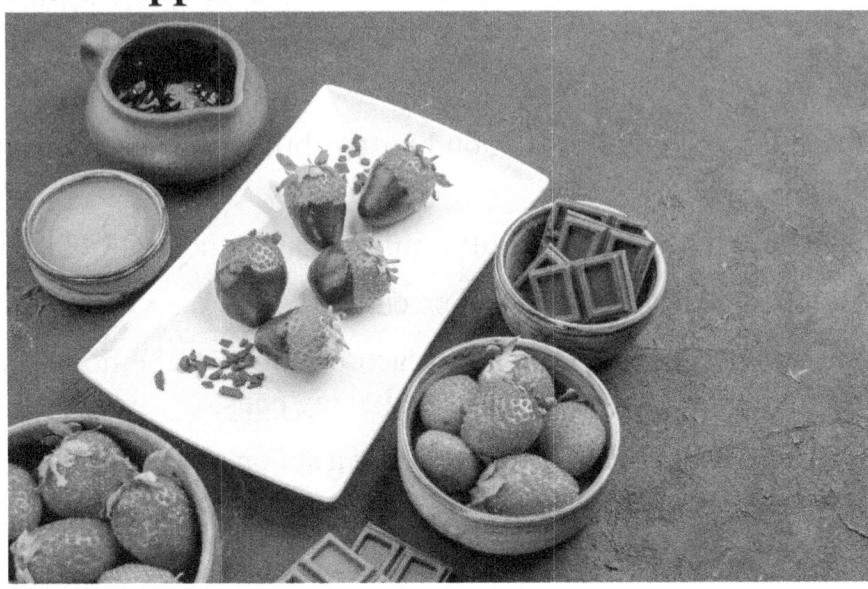

(Servings: 4 | Prep Time: 10 minutes)

Ingredients:

- 1 cup fresh strawberries, washed and dried
- 1/2 cup dark chocolate chips
- 1 teaspoon coconut oil

Instructions:

- In a microwave-safe bowl, combine the dark chocolate chips and coconut oil. Microwave in 30-second intervals, stirring in between, until the chocolate is melted and smooth.
- Dip each strawberry into the melted chocolate, coating about two-thirds of the strawberry.
- Place the dipped strawberries on a parchment-lined tray.
- Let the chocolate harden by refrigerating the tray for about 10 minutes.
- Serve immediately or store in the refrigerator for up to 2 days.

Nutritional Info: Calories: 120kcal | Fat: 8g | Carb: 13g | Fiber: 3g | Sugar: 8g | Protein: 2g

9. Pumpkin Spice Protein Bites

(Servings: 12 | Prep Time: 15 minutes)

Ingredients:

- 1 cup rolled oats
- 1/2 cup pumpkin puree
- 1/4 cup almond butter
- 1/4 cup honey or maple syrup
- 1 teaspoon pumpkin pie spice
- 1/2 cup unsweetened shredded coconut (optional, for rolling)

Instructions:

- In a large mixing bowl, combine the rolled oats, pumpkin puree, almond butter, honey (or maple syrup), and pumpkin pie spice. Mix well until a thick, sticky dough forms.
- Take about 1 tablespoon of the mixture and roll it into a ball using your hands.
- If desired, roll the balls in shredded coconut to coat them.
- Place the protein bites on a plate or baking sheet lined with parchment paper.
- Refrigerate for at least 15 minutes to firm up before serving.
- Store the pumpkin spice protein bites in an airtight container in the refrigerator for up to 1 week.

Nutritional Info: Calories: 110kcal | Fat: 5g | Carb: 15g | Fiber: 2g | Sugar: 7g | Protein: 3g

10. Peanut Butter Banana Bites

(Servings: 4 | Prep Time: 10 minutes)

Ingredients:

- 2 medium ripe bananas, peeled and sliced into 1-inch pieces
- 2 tablespoons peanut butter
- 2 tablespoons unsweetened shredded coconut
- 2 tablespoons chopped peanuts (optional, for garnish)

Instructions:

- Spread peanut butter on one side of each banana slice.
- Sprinkle shredded coconut over the peanut butter on half of the banana slices.
- Top each coconut-covered slice with another banana slice to make a sandwich.
- Press gently to stick the two slices together.

- If desired, roll the edges of the banana bites in chopped peanuts for extra crunch.
- Serve immediately or refrigerate for up to 2 days.

Nutritional Info: Calories: 110kcal | Fat: 5g | Carb: 14g | Fiber: 2g | Sugar: 7g | Protein: 2g

11. Lemon Coconut Bliss Balls

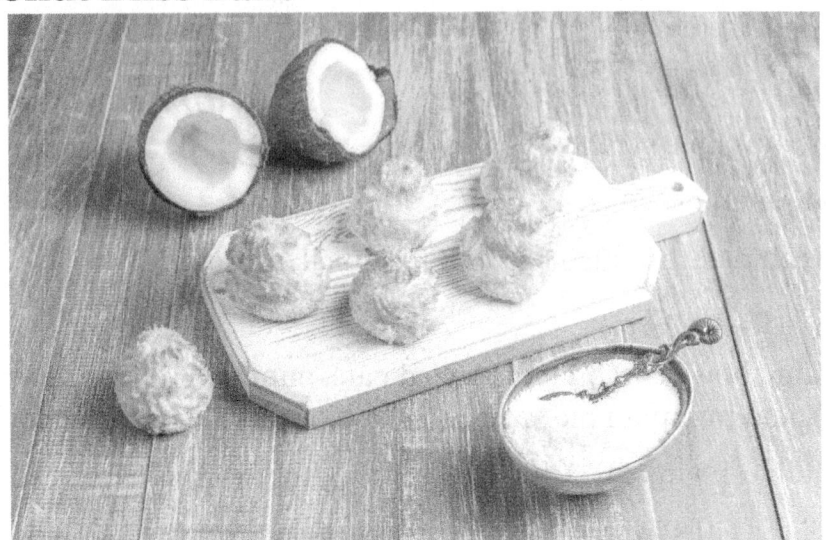

(Servings: 10 | Prep Time: 15 minutes | Total Time: 30 minutes)

Ingredients:

- 1 cup unsweetened shredded coconut, plus extra for rolling
- 1/2 cup raw cashews
- Zest and juice of 1 lemon
- 2 tablespoons honey or maple syrup
- 1 teaspoon vanilla extract

Instructions:

- In a food processor, combine the shredded coconut, cashews, lemon zest, lemon juice, honey (or maple syrup), and vanilla extract.
- Process until the mixture becomes sticky and holds together when pressed with your fingers.
- Take about 1 tablespoon of the mixture and roll it into a ball using your hands.
- Roll each bliss ball in additional shredded coconut to coat.
- Place the bliss balls on a plate or baking sheet lined with parchment paper.
- Refrigerate for at least 15 minutes to firm up before serving.
- Store the lemon coconut bliss balls in an airtight container in the refrigerator for up to 1 week.

Nutritional Info: Calories: 130kcal | Fat: 10g | Carb: 9g | Fiber: 2g | Sugar: 5g | Protein: 2g

12. Cinnamon Apple Chips

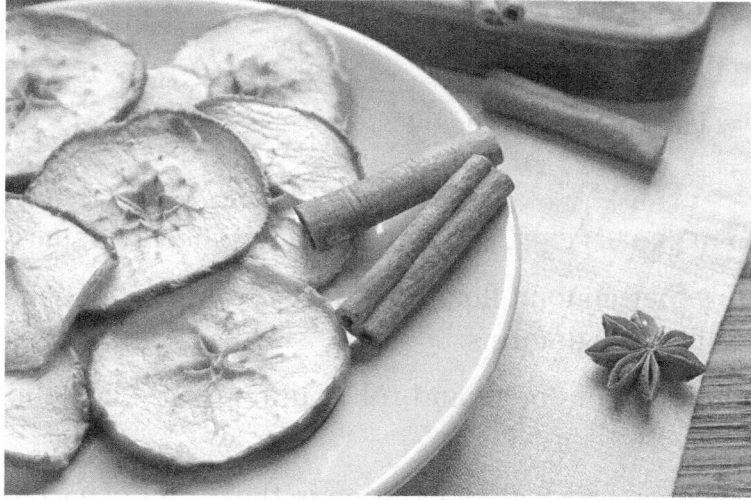

(Servings: 4 | Prep Time: 10 minutes | Total Time: 2 hours 20 minutes)

Ingredients:

- 2 large apples (such as Fuji or Honeycrisp)
- 1 teaspoon ground cinnamon
- 1 teaspoon granulated sugar (optional)

Instructions:

- Preheat the oven to 200°F (95°C). Line two baking sheets with parchment paper.
- Slice the apples thinly using a sharp knife or a mandoline slicer.
- In a large mixing bowl, toss the apple slices with cinnamon and sugar (if using), making sure they are evenly coated.
- Arrange the apple slices in a single layer on the prepared baking sheets.
- Bake in the preheated oven for 2 to 2.5 hours, or until the apple chips are crispy and no longer moist.
- Allow the apple chips to cool completely before serving.
- Store the cinnamon apple chips in an airtight container at room temperature for up to 1 week.

Nutritional Info: Calories: 60kcal | Fat: 0.3g | Carbohydrates: 15g | Fiber: 3g | Sugar: 11g | Protein: 0.3g

13. Raspberry Almond Thumbprint Cookies

(Servings: 12 | Prep Time: 15 minutes | Cook Time: 12 minutes)

Ingredients:

- 1 cup almond flour

- 1/4 cup coconut oil, softened
- 2 tablespoons maple syrup or honey
- 1/2 teaspoon almond extract
- 1/4 cup raspberry jam (no added sugar)

Instructions:

- Preheat the oven to 350°F (175°C) and line a baking sheet with parchment paper.
- In a bowl, mix together almond flour, softened coconut oil, maple syrup (or honey), and almond extract until a dough forms.
- Take about 1 tablespoon of dough and roll it into a ball. Place the balls on the prepared baking sheet.
- Use your thumb to create a small indentation in the center of each cookie.
- Fill each indentation with raspberry jam.
- Bake in the preheated oven for about 12 minutes, or until the cookies are golden brown around the edges.
- Allow the cookies to cool on the baking sheet for a few minutes before transferring them to a wire rack to cool completely.
- Store the raspberry almond thumbprint cookies in an airtight container at room temperature for up to 5 days.

Nutritional Info: Calories: 110kcal | Fat: 8g | Carb: 8g | Fiber: 2g | Sugar: 4g | Protein: 2g

14. No-Bake Oatmeal Energy Bars

(Servings: 12 | Prep Time: 15 minutes | Total Time: 1 hour 15 minutes)

Ingredients:

- 1 cup rolled oats
- 1/2 cup almond butter
- 1/4 cup honey or maple syrup
- 1/4 cup unsweetened shredded coconut
- 1/4 cup chopped almonds
- 1/4 cup dried cranberries (or other dried fruits)

Instructions:

- In a large mixing bowl, combine rolled oats, almond butter, honey (or maple syrup), shredded coconut, chopped almonds, and dried cranberries.
- Mix well until all the ingredients are evenly distributed and the mixture sticks together when pressed.

- Line a baking dish with parchment paper.
- Press the oat mixture into the baking dish, smoothing the top with a spatula or your hands.
- Refrigerate for at least 1 hour to firm up before cutting into bars.
- Cut into bars or squares and serve.
- Store the oatmeal energy bars in an airtight container in the refrigerator for up to 1 week.

Nutritional Info: Calories: 170kcal | Fat: 10g | Carb: 17g | Fiber: 3g | Sugar: 8g | Protein: 4g

15. Chocolate Avocado Pudding
(Servings: 4 | Prep Time: 10 minutes | Total Time: 2 hours 10 minutes)

Ingredients:
- 2 ripe avocados, peeled and pitted
- 1/4 cup unsweetened cocoa powder
- 1/4 cup honey or maple syrup
- 1/4 cup almond milk (or any milk of your choice)
- 1 teaspoon vanilla extract
- Pinch of salt

Instructions:
- In a blender or food processor, combine the avocados, cocoa powder, honey (or maple syrup), almond milk, vanilla extract, and salt.
- Blend until smooth and creamy, scraping down the sides as needed.
- Taste and adjust sweetness if desired.
- Transfer the pudding to serving cups or bowls.
- Refrigerate for at least 2 hours to chill and set before serving.
- Serve chilled, garnished with fresh berries or a sprinkle of cocoa powder if desired.

Nutritional Info: Calories: 180kcal | Fat: 10g | Carb: 25g | Fiber: 7g | Sugar: 15g | Protein: 3g

60-Day Meal Plan: 16:8 (16 hours fasting, 8 hours eating)

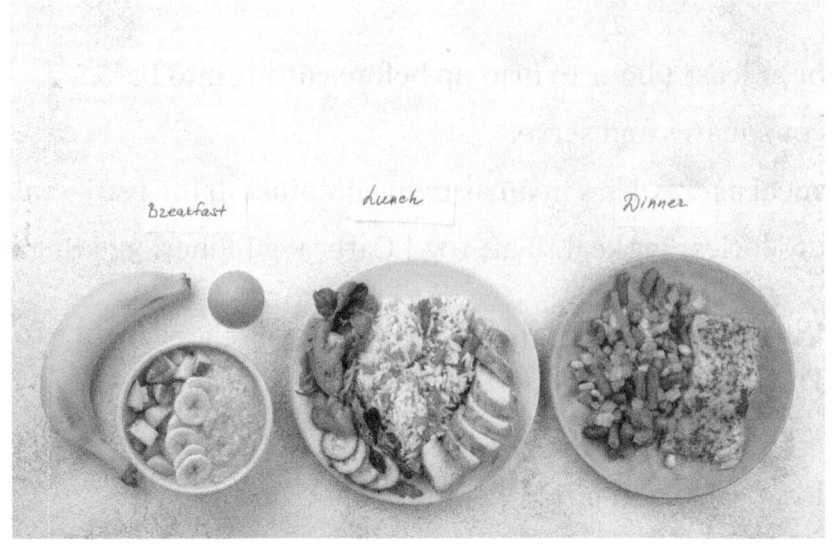

Day 1

Eating Window: 10 AM - 6 PM

Breakfast: Poached Eggs & Avocado Toasts

(Avocado provides healthy fats and fiber, promoting satiety and heart health)

Snack: Roasted Cauliflower "Popcorn"

Lunch: Warm Roasted Vegetable Farro Salad

(Farro is a nutritious whole grain rich in protein and fiber)

Snack: Lemon Coconut Bliss Balls

Dinner: Cajun Potato, Prawn/Shrimp, and Avocado Salad

Day 2

Eating Window: 11 AM - 7 PM

Breakfast: Greek Yogurt Parfait with Berries and Almonds

(Greek yogurt is an excellent source of protein and probiotics for gut health)

Snack: Cinnamon Apple Chips

Lunch: Roasted Broccoli with Lemon Garlic & Toasted Pine Nuts

Snack: Spicy Chocolate Keto Fat Bombs

(These fat bombs can satisfy sweet cravings without spiking blood sugar levels)

Dinner: Cauliflower Rice Stir-Fry with Tofu and Vegetables

Day 3

Eating Window: 12 PM - 8 PM

Breakfast: Almond Flour Pancakes with Sugar-Free Syrup

(Use sugar-free syrup to reduce added sugars in your breakfast)

Snack: Frozen Strawberry-Chocolate Greek Yogurt

Lunch: Lentil Veggie Burgers

Snack: Peanut Butter Banana Bites

(Peanut butter adds a protein boost and healthy fats to the snack)

Dinner: Lemon Garlic Shrimp and Asparagus Stir-Fry

Day 4

Eating Window: 10 AM - 6 PM

Breakfast: Quinoa Breakfast Bowl with Nuts and Seeds

(Nuts and seeds are rich in essential nutrients and provide a satisfying crunch to the bowl)

Snack: Mango and Passionfruit Roulade

Lunch: Baked Mahi Mahi

Snack: Pumpkin Spice Protein Bites

(Pumpkin spice bites offer a protein-rich snack to keep you full longer)

Dinner: Moroccan Chickpea Stew with Quinoa

Day 5

Eating Window: 11 AM - 7 PM

Breakfast: Green Smoothie with Spinach, Kale, and Pineapple

(The green smoothie provides a nutrient-packed start to the day)

Snack: Citrus Dark Chocolate Mousse

Lunch: BBQ Chicken Tostadas

Snack: Peanut Butter Cookies

(Opt for natural peanut butter with no added sugars or oils)

Dinner: Grilled Lemon Herb Salmon

Day 6

Eating Window: 12 PM - 8 PM

Breakfast: Zucchini and Spinach Egg Muffins

(These egg muffins are easy to make and can be refrigerated for a quick breakfast)

Snack: No-Bake Oatmeal Energy Bars
Lunch: Teriyaki Tofu and Vegetable Skewers
Snack: Lemon Herb Baked Cod with Steamed Green Beans
(Baking the cod preserves its moisture and nutrients)
Dinner: Ratatouille with Herbed Quinoa

Day 7
Eating Window: 10 AM - 6 PM
Breakfast: Blueberry Protein Smoothie
(Add protein powder to boost the protein content of the smoothie)
Snack: Roasted Cauliflower "Popcorn"
Lunch: Shrimp Diablo Spaghetti
Snack: Peanut Butter Cookies
Dinner: Grilled Steak with Chimichurri Sauce and Roasted Sweet Potatoes

Tips for Women Over 60
- **Stay Hydrated:** As we age, our sense of thirst may decrease, so it's essential to drink enough water throughout the day. Aim for at least 8 glasses of water daily.
- **Choose Nutrient-Dense Foods:** Focus on foods that provide essential nutrients, such as fruits, vegetables, lean proteins, and whole grains.
- **Include Calcium-Rich Foods:** Calcium is crucial for bone health. Incorporate sources like dairy, leafy greens, or fortified alternatives.

Shopping Advice
- Opt for fresh produce and lean proteins to create nutritious meals.
- Choose whole grains like quinoa and farro for added fiber and nutrients.
- Stock up on healthy fats like avocado, nuts, and olive oil for cooking and snacks.
- Look for sugar-free or low-sugar options for desserts and snacks.
- Buy frozen fruits and vegetables for smoothies and quick meal preparation.

Day 8
Eating Window: 12 PM - 6 PM
Breakfast: Greek Yogurt Parfait with Berries and Almonds
Snack: Cinnamon Apple Chips
Lunch: Teriyaki Tofu and Vegetable Skewers
Snack: Spicy Chocolate Keto Fat Bombs

Dinner: Baked Parmesan Tilapia Delight

Day 9
Eating Window: 1 PM - 7 PM
Breakfast: Quinoa Breakfast Bowl with Nuts and Seeds
Snack: Dark Chocolate Dipped Strawberries
Lunch: Moroccan Chickpea Stew with Quinoa
Snack: Roasted Cauliflower "Popcorn"
Dinner: Grilled Lemon Herb Salmon

Day 10
Eating Window: 2 PM - 8 PM
Breakfast: Zucchini and Spinach Egg Muffins
Snack: Almond Butter Chocolate Chip Cookies
Lunch: Buffalo Chicken Sandwich with Blue Cheese Slaw
Snack: Lemon Coconut Bliss Balls
Dinner: Vegetable Turkey Meatloaf with Balsamic Glaze

Day 11
Eating Window: 12 PM - 6 PM
Breakfast: Chia Seed Pudding with Mixed Berries
Snack: Frozen Strawberry-Chocolate Greek Yogurt
Lunch: Lemon Garlic Shrimp and Asparagus Stir-Fry
Snack: Peanut Butter Banana Bites
Dinner: Cauliflower Pizza Crust

Day 12
Eating Window: 1 PM - 7 PM
Breakfast: Blueberry Protein Smoothie
Snack: Raspberry Almond Thumbprint Cookies
Lunch: Oriental Turkey Burger
Snack: No-Bake Oatmeal Energy Bars
Dinner: Rustic Shepherd's Pie

Day 13

Eating Window: 2 PM - 8 PM

Breakfast: Baked Potato

Snack: Mango and Passionfruit Roulade

Lunch: BBQ Chicken Tostadas

Snack: Citrus Dark Chocolate Mousse

Dinner: Sweet Potato Curry With Spinach And Chickpeas

Day 14

Eating Window: 12 PM - 6 PM

Breakfast: Poached Eggs & Avocado Toasts

Snack: Peanut Butter Cookies

Lunch: Greek Chicken Souvlaki with Tzatziki Sauce

Snack: Chocolate Avocado Pudding

Dinner: Shredded Brussels Sprouts with Bacon and Onions

Tips for Women Over 60

- **Prioritize Protein:** Including enough protein in your meals can help preserve muscle mass and support overall health.
- **Listen to Your Body:** Pay attention to hunger cues and eat until you feel satisfied. Avoid overeating or restricting calories too much.
- **Be Mindful of Sodium:** Watch your sodium intake, as excess salt may contribute to bloating and other health issues.

Shopping Advice

- Purchase tofu, tempeh, or lean meats for protein sources.
- Choose plenty of leafy greens and colorful vegetables for nutrient-packed meals.
- Consider using herbs and spices to enhance the flavors of your dishes without added salt.
- Stock up on frozen fruits and vegetables for convenience and to reduce waste.
- Include a variety of nuts and seeds for snacking and to add crunch to salads.

Day 15

Eating Window: 1 PM - 7 PM

Breakfast: Baked Mahi Mahi

Snack: Roasted Cauliflower "Popcorn"

Lunch: Roasted Broccoli with Lemon Garlic & Toasted Pine Nuts

Snack: Cinnamon Apple Chips
Dinner: Eggplant and Chickpea Coconut Curry with Brown Rice

Day 16
Eating Window: 12 PM - 6 PM
Breakfast: French Vanilla Almond Granola
Snack: Mango and Passionfruit Roulade
Lunch: Teriyaki Tofu and Vegetable Skewers
Snack: Raspberry Almond Thumbprint Cookies
Dinner: Grilled Steak with Chimichurri Sauce and Roasted Sweet Potatoes

Day 17
Eating Window: 1 PM - 7 PM
Breakfast: Baked Potato
Snack: Peanut Butter Cookies
Lunch: Ratatouille with Herbed Quinoa
Snack: Citrus Dark Chocolate Mousse
Dinner: Spicy Spanish Tomato Baked Eggs

Day 18
Eating Window: 2 PM - 8 PM
Breakfast: Green Smoothie with Spinach, Kale, and Pineapple
Snack: Dark Chocolate Dipped Strawberries
Lunch: BBQ Chicken Tostadas
Snack: No-Bake Oatmeal Energy Bars
Dinner: Cauliflower Pizza Crust

Day 19
Eating Window: 12 PM - 6 PM
Breakfast: Poached Eggs & Avocado Toasts
Snack: Mango and Passionfruit Roulade
Lunch: Shrimp Diablo Spaghetti
Snack: Almond Butter Chocolate Chip Cookies
Dinner: Italian Chicken

Day 20

Eating Window: 1 PM - 7 PM

Breakfast: Chia Seed Pudding with Mixed Berries

Snack: Frozen Strawberry-Chocolate Greek Yogurt

Lunch: Moroccan Chickpea Stew with Quinoa

Snack: Roasted Cauliflower "Popcorn"

Dinner: Sweet Potato Curry With Spinach And Chickpeas

Day 21

Eating Window: 2 PM - 8 PM

Breakfast: Zucchini and Spinach Egg Muffins

Snack: Peanut Butter Banana Bites

Lunch: Lemon Garlic Shrimp and Asparagus Stir-Fry

Snack: Raspberry Almond Thumbprint Cookies

Dinner: Vegetable Turkey Meatloaf with Balsamic Glaze

Tips for Women Over 60

- **Embrace Hobbies:** Engage in hobbies or activities that bring you joy and fulfillment. It's essential for mental well-being.
- **Manage Stress:** Practice relaxation techniques like deep breathing, meditation, or spending time in nature to reduce stress levels.
- **Prioritize Sleep:** Aim for 7-9 hours of quality sleep each night to support overall health and well-being.
- **Social Connection:** Stay connected with friends and loved ones. Social interactions can have positive effects on mental health.

Shopping Advice

- Choose organic and non-GMO ingredients whenever possible.
- Opt for lean protein sources like chicken, turkey, and fish.
- Buy whole grains such as quinoa, brown rice, and oats for fiber-rich meals.
- Don't forget to stock up on a variety of fresh fruits and vegetables for balanced nutrition.
- Check your pantry for necessary spices and condiments to add flavor to your dishes.

Day 22

Eating Window: 12 PM - 6 PM

Breakfast: Greek Yogurt Parfait with Berries and Almonds

Snack: Lemon Coconut Bliss Balls
Lunch: Cauliflower Rice Stir-Fry with Tofu and Vegetables
Snack: Mango and Passionfruit Roulade
Dinner: Rustic Shepherd's Pie

Day 23
Eating Window: 1 PM - 7 PM
Breakfast: Almond Flour Pancakes with Sugar-Free Syrup
Snack: Citrus Dark Chocolate Mousse
Lunch: Spinach and Mushroom Stuffed Portobello Mushrooms
Snack: Spicy Chocolate Keto Fat Bombs
Dinner: Shredded Brussels Sprouts with Bacon and Onions

Day 24
Eating Window: 2 PM - 8 PM
Breakfast: Baked Mahi Mahi
Snack: Roasted Cauliflower "Popcorn"
Lunch: Cauliflower Pizza Crust
Snack: Cinnamon Apple Chips
Dinner: Eggplant and Chickpea Coconut Curry with Brown Rice

Day 25
Eating Window: 12 PM - 6 PM
Breakfast: Poached Eggs & Avocado Toasts
Snack: Peanut Butter Cookies
Lunch: Baked Parmesan Tilapia Delight
Snack: No-Bake Oatmeal Energy Bars
Dinner: Lemon Herb Baked Cod with Steamed Green Beans

Day 26
Eating Window: 1 PM - 7 PM
Breakfast: Green Smoothie with Spinach, Kale, and Pineapple
Snack: Dark Chocolate Dipped Strawberries
Lunch: Quinoa Stuffed Bell Peppers with Black Beans and Avocado
Snack: Almond Butter Chocolate Chip Cookies

Dinner: Cajun Potato, Prawn/Shrimp, and Avocado Salad

Day 27

Eating Window: 2 PM - 8 P

Breakfast: Chia Seed Pudding with Mixed Berries

Snack: Lemon Coconut Bliss Balls

Lunch: Mediterranean Zoodle Bowl with Olives and Feta

Snack: Frozen Strawberry-Chocolate Greek Yogurt

Dinner: Vegetable Frittata with Turmeric and Herbs

Day 28

Eating Window: 12 PM - 6 PM

Breakfast: French Vanilla Almond Granola

Snack: Citrus Dark Chocolate Mousse

Lunch: Buffalo Chicken Sandwich with Blue Cheese Slaw

Snack: Cinnamon Apple Chips

Dinner: Moroccan Chickpea Stew with Quinoa

Tips for Women Over 60

- **Be Mindful of Sugars:** Limit added sugars in your meals and snacks to support blood sugar levels and overall health.
- **Nutrient-Dense Choices:** Choose nutrient-dense foods to ensure you get essential vitamins and minerals in your diet.
- **Hydration with Herbal Teas:** Stay hydrated with herbal teas like chamomile, peppermint, or ginger, which offer additional health benefits.

Day 29

Eating Window: 1 PM - 7 PM

Breakfast: Smoked Salmon and Avocado Wrap

Snack: Roasted Cauliflower "Popcorn"

Lunch: Roasted Broccoli with Lemon Garlic & Toasted Pine Nuts

Snack: Raspberry Almond Thumbprint Cookies

Dinner: Baked Eggplant Parmesan with Mixed Greens Salad

Day 30
Eating Window: 2 PM - 8 PM
Breakfast: Zucchini and Cheese Scrambled Eggs
Snack: Dark Chocolate Dipped Strawberries
Lunch: Teriyaki Tofu and Vegetable Skewers
Snack: Almond Butter Chocolate Chip Cookies
Dinner: Cauliflower Pizza Crust

Day 31
Eating Window: 12 PM - 6 PM
Breakfast: Baked Potato
Snack: Peanut Butter Banana Bites
Lunch: Asian Sesame Chicken Salad
Snack: No-Bake Oatmeal Energy Bars
Dinner: Teriyaki Salmon with Sesame Broccoli

Day 32
Eating Window: 1 PM - 7 PM
Breakfast: Egg Scramble with Sweet Potatoes
Snack: Lemon Coconut Bliss Balls
Lunch: Shredded Brussels Sprouts with Bacon and Onions
Snack: Spicy Chocolate Keto Fat Bombs
Dinner: Quinoa Stuffed Bell Peppers with Black Beans and Avocado

Day 33
Eating Window: 2 PM - 8 PM
Breakfast: Green Smoothie with Spinach, Kale, and Pineapple
Snack: Citrus Dark Chocolate Mousse
Lunch: Mediterranean Zoodle Bowl with Olives and Feta
Snack: Frozen Strawberry-Chocolate Greek Yogurt
Dinner: Vegetable Frittata with Turmeric and Herbs

Day 34
Eating Window: 12 PM - 6 PM
Breakfast: Poached Eggs & Avocado Toasts

Snack: Peanut Butter Cookies
Lunch: Italian Chicken
Snack: Cinnamon Apple Chips
Dinner: Eggplant and Chickpea Coconut Curry with Brown Rice

Day 35
Eating Window: 1 PM - 7 PM
Breakfast: French Vanilla Almond Granola
Snack: Lemon Coconut Bliss Balls
Lunch: Cauliflower Rice Stir-Fry with Tofu and Vegetables
Snack: Mango and Passionfruit Roulade
Dinner: Rustic Shepherd's Pie

Day 36
Eating Window: 2 PM - 8 PM
Breakfast: Chia Seed Pudding with Mixed Berries
Snack: Dark Chocolate Dipped Strawberries
Lunch: Zucchini Noodles with Pesto and Cherry Tomatoes
Snack: Almond Butter Chocolate Chip Cookies
Dinner: Cajun Potato, Prawn/Shrimp, and Avocado Salad

Day 37
Eating Window: 12 PM - 6 PM
Breakfast: Smoked Salmon and Avocado Wrap
Snack: Citrus Dark Chocolate Mousse
Lunch: Baked Mahi Mahi
Snack: Cinnamon Apple Chips
Dinner: Ratatouille with Herbed Quinoa

Day 38
Eating Window: 1 PM - 7 PM
Breakfast: Zucchini and Cheese Scrambled Eggs
Snack: Roasted Cauliflower "Popcorn"
Lunch: Lentil Veggie Burgers
Snack: Raspberry Almond Thumbprint Cookies

Dinner: Vegetable Turkey Meatloaf with Balsamic Glaze

Day 39
Eating Window: 2 PM - 8 PM
Breakfast: Green Smoothie with Spinach, Kale, and Pineapple
Snack: Peanut Butter Cookies
Lunch: BBQ Chicken Tostadas
Snack: No-Bake Oatmeal Energy Bars
Dinner: Spinach and Mushroom Stuffed Portobello Mushrooms

Day 40
Eating Window: 12 PM - 6 PM
Breakfast: Poached Eggs & Avocado Toasts
Snack: Lemon Coconut Bliss Balls
Lunch: Shrimp Diablo Spaghetti
Snack: Mango and Passionfruit Roulade
Dinner: Baked Parmesan Tilapia Delight

Day 41
Eating Window: 1 PM - 7 PM
Breakfast: Chia Seed Pudding with Mixed Berries
Snack: Dark Chocolate Dipped Strawberries
Lunch: Lemon Herb Baked Cod with Steamed Green Beans
Snack: Almond Butter Chocolate Chip Cookies
Dinner: Sweet Potato Curry With Spinach And Chickpeas

Day 42
Eating Window: 2 PM - 8 PM
Breakfast: Zucchini and Spinach Egg Muffins
Snack: Citrus Dark Chocolate Mousse
Lunch: Teriyaki Tofu and Vegetable Skewers
Snack: Cinnamon Apple Chips
Dinner: Rustic Shepherd's Pie

Day 43

Eating Window: 12 PM - 6 PM

Breakfast: Greek Yogurt Parfait with Berries and Almonds

Snack: Peanut Butter Banana Bites

Lunch: Grilled Lemon Herb Salmon

Snack: Roasted Cauliflower "Popcorn"

Dinner: Moroccan Chickpea Stew with Quinoa

Day 44

Eating Window: 1 PM - 7 PM

Breakfast: Baked Potato

Snack: Lemon Coconut Bliss Balls

Lunch: Cauliflower Pizza Crust

Snack: Frozen Strawberry-Chocolate Greek Yogurt

Dinner: Ratatouille with Herbed Quinoa

Day 45

Eating Window: 2 PM - 8 PM

Breakfast: Egg Scramble with Sweet Potatoes

Snack: Dark Chocolate Dipped Strawberries

Lunch: Lemon Garlic Shrimp and Asparagus Stir-Fry

Snack: Almond Butter Chocolate Chip Cookies

Dinner: Grilled Steak with Chimichurri Sauce and Roasted Sweet Potatoes

Tips for Women Over 60 & Shopping Advice

- **Choose Healthy Fats:** Include healthy fats from sources like avocados, nuts, seeds, and olive oil. These fats support brain function and help with nutrient absorption.
- **Buy Frozen Fruits and Vegetables:** Keep frozen fruits and vegetables on hand for quick and convenient additions to smoothies, stir-fries, and meals.
- **Moderate Caffeine Intake:** Limit caffeinated beverages to avoid disturbances in sleep patterns.
- **Stock Up on Herbs and Spices:** Enhance the flavor of your meals with herbs and spices like turmeric, garlic, basil, and oregano. They provide antioxidants and may have anti-inflammatory properties.
- **Read Labels:** When buying packaged foods, read the nutrition labels carefully. Look for products with lower added sugars, sodium, and unhealthy fats.

Day 46
Eating Window: 2 PM - 8 PM
Breakfast: Green Smoothie with Spinach, Kale, and Pineapple
Snack: Peanut Butter Cookies
Lunch: BBQ Chicken Tostadas
Snack: No-Bake Oatmeal Energy Bars
Dinner: Spinach and Mushroom Stuffed Portobello Mushrooms

Day 47
Eating Window: 12 PM - 6 PM
Breakfast: Poached Eggs & Avocado Toasts
Snack: Citrus Dark Chocolate Mousse
Lunch: Mediterranean Zoodle Bowl with Olives and Feta
Snack: Mango and Passionfruit Roulade
Dinner: Quinoa Stuffed Bell Peppers with Black Beans and Avocado

Day 48
Eating Window: 2 PM - 8 PM
Breakfast: Egg Scramble with Sweet Potatoes
Snack: Dark Chocolate Dipped Strawberries
Lunch: Lemon Garlic Shrimp and Asparagus Stir-Fry
Snack: Almond Butter Chocolate Chip Cookies
Dinner: Grilled Steak with Chimichurri Sauce and Roasted Sweet Potatoes

Day 49
Eating Window: 1 PM - 7 PM
Breakfast: Baked Potato
Snack: Lemon Coconut Bliss Balls
Lunch: Cauliflower Pizza Crust
Snack: Frozen Strawberry-Chocolate Greek Yogurt
Dinner: Ratatouille with Herbed Quinoa

Day 50
Eating Window: 12 PM - 6 PM
Breakfast: Greek Yogurt Parfait with Berries and Almonds

Snack: Peanut Butter Banana Bites
Lunch: Grilled Lemon Herb Salmon
Snack: Roasted Cauliflower "Popcorn"
Dinner: Moroccan Chickpea Stew with Quinoa

Day 51
Eating Window: 2 PM - 8 PM
Breakfast: Zucchini and Spinach Egg Muffins
Snack: Citrus Dark Chocolate Mousse
Lunch: Teriyaki Tofu and Vegetable Skewers
Snack: Cinnamon Apple Chips
Dinner: Rustic Shepherd's Pie

Day 52
Eating Window: 1 PM - 7 PM
Breakfast: Chia Seed Pudding with Mixed Berries
Snack: Dark Chocolate Dipped Strawberries
Lunch: Lemon Herb Baked Cod with Steamed Green Beans
Snack: Almond Butter Chocolate Chip Cookies
Dinner: Sweet Potato Curry With Spinach And Chickpeas

Day 53
Eating Window: 12 PM - 6 PM
Breakfast: Poached Eggs & Avocado Toasts
Snack: Lemon Coconut Bliss Balls
Lunch: Shrimp Diablo Spaghetti
Snack: Mango and Passionfruit Roulade
Dinner: Baked Parmesan Tilapia Delight

Day 54
Eating Window: 1 PM - 7 PM
Breakfast: Zucchini and Cheese Scrambled Eggs
Snack: Roasted Cauliflower "Popcorn"
Lunch: Baked Mahi Mahi
Snack: Raspberry Almond Thumbprint Cookies

Dinner: Vegetable Turkey Meatloaf with Balsamic Glaze

Day 55
Eating Window: 2 PM - 8 PM
Breakfast: Green Smoothie with Spinach, Kale, and Pineapple
Snack: Peanut Butter Cookies
Lunch: BBQ Chicken Tostadas
Snack: No-Bake Oatmeal Energy Bars
Dinner: Spinach and Mushroom Stuffed Portobello Mushrooms

Day 56
Eating Window: 12 PM - 6 PM
Breakfast: Poached Eggs & Avocado Toasts
Snack: Citrus Dark Chocolate Mousse
Lunch: Mediterranean Zoodle Bowl with Olives and Feta
Snack: Mango and Passionfruit Roulade
Dinner: Quinoa Stuffed Bell Peppers with Black Beans and Avocado

Day 57
Eating Window: 2 PM - 8 PM
Breakfast: Zucchini and Spinach Egg Muffins
Snack: Citrus Dark Chocolate Mousse
Lunch: Teriyaki Tofu and Vegetable Skewers
Snack: Cinnamon Apple Chips
Dinner: Rustic Shepherd's Pie

Day 58
Eating Window: 1 PM - 7 PM
Breakfast: Chia Seed Pudding with Mixed Berries
Snack: Dark Chocolate Dipped Strawberries
Lunch: Lemon Herb Baked Cod with Steamed Green Beans
Snack: Almond Butter Chocolate Chip Cookies
Dinner: Sweet Potato Curry With Spinach And Chickpeas

Day 59

Eating Window: 12 PM - 6 PM

Breakfast: Poached Eggs & Avocado Toasts

Snack: Lemon Coconut Bliss Balls

Lunch: Shrimp Diablo Spaghetti

Snack: Mango and Passionfruit Roulade

Dinner: Baked Parmesan Tilapia Delight

Day 60

Eating Window: 2 PM - 8 PM

Breakfast: Green Smoothie with Spinach, Kale, and Pineapple

Snack: Peanut Butter Cookies

Lunch: BBQ Chicken Tostadas

Snack: No-Bake Oatmeal Energy Bars

Dinner: Spinach and Mushroom Stuffed Portobello Mushrooms

Tips for Women Over 60 & Shopping Advice

- **Go for Lean Proteins:** Select lean protein sources like chicken, turkey, fish, tofu, legumes, and low-fat dairy to support muscle health and maintenance.

- **Incorporate Plant-Based Proteins:** Explore plant-based protein sources such as lentils, chickpeas, quinoa, and nuts to diversify your protein intake and promote heart health.

- **Choose Low-Sodium Options:** Opt for low-sodium versions of canned or packaged foods to reduce sodium intake.

- **Meal Prep:** Prepare meals in advance to make it easier to stick to your meal plan and avoid impulsive food choices.

- **Avoid Sugary Beverages:** Limit sugary drinks like soda and fruit juices, and opt for water or herbal teas instead.

Guided Intermittent Fasting Tracker

Name:

Start Date of Tracking:

Intermittent Fasting Goal:

Fasting Window

Record the start and end times of your daily fasting window. You can also note any variations in fasting duration or days when you followed a different fasting window.

Day 1	**Day 2**
Fasting Start Time:	Fasting Start Time:
Fasting End Time:	Fasting End Time:
Notes:	Notes:

...

Nutrition Intake

Log the meals and snacks you consume during the eating window. Pay attention to portion sizes and the quality of foods you choose.

Day 1	**Day 2**
Meal 1:	Meal 1:
Meal 2:	Meal 2:
Snack:	Snack:
Notes:	Notes:

...

Non-Scale Victories

Every day, write down the non-scale victories you experienced thanks to intermittent fasting. These could include improved digestion, reduced cravings, enhanced focus, or healthier skin.

Day 1

Non-Scale Victory:

Notes:

...

Day 2

Non-Scale Victory:

Notes:

Energy and Well-being

Monitor your energy levels and overall well-being throughout the day. Take note of any variations or changes you noticed.

Day 1

Energy Levels:

General Well-being:

Notes:

Day 2

Energy Levels:

General Well-being:

Notes:

...

Physical Changes

Occasionally, take time to evaluate any physical changes. These may include weight loss, measurements, or body composition.

Day 1	**Day 2**
Weight:	Weight:
Measurements:	Measurements:
Body Composition:	Body Composition:
Notes:	Notes

...

Guided Roadmap for Intermittent Fasting

These guides will help the reader track their intermittent fasting progress in a structured and mindful way. Remind them to be patient with themselves, as every body responds differently. The key is to tailor intermittent fasting to their individual needs and experiment until they find the best routine for their journey.

Step 1: Choose Your Tracker

Select the tracking method that suits you best: pen and paper, mobile app, or smartwatch/fitness tracker.

Step 2: Clear Goals

Clearly define your intermittent fasting goals, such as weight loss, improved energy, or better mental clarity.

Step 3: Fasting Windows

Record the start and end times of your daily fasting window and experiment with different fasting windows to find the one that works best for you.

Step 4: Mindful Eating

Monitor what you eat during the eating windows, ensuring you make nutritious and balanced choices.

Step 5: Non-Scale Victories

Recognize victories unrelated to the scale, such as better sleep, reduced heartburn, or an improved mood.

Step 6: Energy and Well-being

Be mindful of your energy levels throughout the day and how intermittent fasting impacts your overall well-being.

Step 7: Physical Changes

Occasionally evaluate any physical changes, but remember that progress may be gradual and vary from person to person.

Step 8: Reflection and Adaptation

Weekly, reflect on your progress and adapt your intermittent fasting routine based on results and personal needs.

Step 9: Celebrate Success

Celebrate your successes and small victories along the intermittent fasting journey to keep motivation high.

Conclusion

This unique combination of books ("Intermittent Fasting for Beginners" and "Intermittent Fasting for Women Over 60") provides a comprehensive approach to intermittent fasting, tailored specifically for beginners and women over 60, ensuring that both groups can embrace the incredible benefits of this transformative dietary practice. In "Intermittent Fasting for Beginners," we delved into the fundamental principles of intermittent fasting. You gained a clear understanding of the various intermittent fasting methods, including the 16/8, 5:2, and Eat-Stop-Eat approaches, empowering you to choose the one that aligns best with your lifestyle and goals. We discussed the health benefits of intermittent fasting, such as improved weight management, enhanced metabolic health, and increased longevity. Moreover, we addressed the potential risks and misconceptions surrounding intermittent fasting, ensuring you can embark on this journey with confidence and safety. "Intermittent Fasting for Women Over 60" took the journey a step further, catering exclusively to the unique needs of women over 60. This book recognized the distinctive health considerations that come with age and offered safe and effective exercises that promote strength, balance, and overall well-being. Our specially curated meal plan, spanning 60 days, ensures that women over 60 can enjoy delicious and nutritious recipes designed to support their specific nutritional needs and complement their intermittent fasting regimen. Throughout both books, we emphasized the importance of a holistic approach to health and wellness. We encouraged you to listen to your body, embrace self-care practices, and celebrate non-scale victories, fostering a positive mindset that extends beyond physical changes. We recognize that embarking on a new dietary journey can be both exciting and challenging, and that's why we provided practical tips and advice at every step of the way. From mindful eating to tracking your progress, from adapting the fasting routine to celebrating successes, we aimed to empower you with the knowledge and tools to make intermittent fasting a sustainable and fulfilling lifestyle choice. Remember, intermittent fasting is not just a diet – it's a journey of self-discovery and empowerment. As you continue along this path, embrace the process, and be patient with yourself. Each individual's experience will be unique, and what matters most is finding an intermittent fasting routine that complements your life and brings you joy.

Made in United States
North Haven, CT
27 February 2024

49271249R00070